Acupuncture and Translocation

an overlooked aspect of medicine, life and spirituality

A treatise on the phenomenon of Translocation

Understood through
Anthroposophy

First edition 2019

By

Are Simeon Thoresen D.V.M.

Acupuncture and Translocation

an overlooked aspect of medicine, life and spirituality

A treatise on the phenomenon of Translocation

Understood through
Anthroposophy

First edition 2019
By
Are Simeon Thoresen D.V.M.

Dedicated to All
Who Seek to Heal and Understand

For questions on the rights of this book please contact:

Are Thoresen
Leikvollgata 31
N-3213 Sandefjord
Email: arethore@online.no

Remark: The author takes no responsibility for the practical use of the methods described in this book.

This book aims to give readers, professional and lay, an understanding of the *spiritual* foundations of alternative medicine, philosophy, principles and practice.

Printed version;
ISBN: 9781080914968

Published by Kindle Books

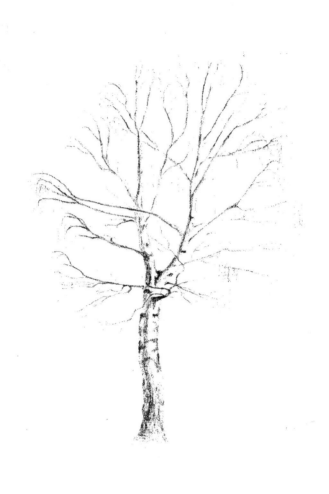

In our physical world I have a strong impression that most of our work and what we do is changing or moving things around. It seems sometimes that our whole life is about translocating things from "A" to "B", repairing or changing, growing food, eating food, discharging it and finally rebuilding it and transforming it through compost.

But, it can also be translocated through the waste water and the sewers, ending up in hurting life.

And as here below, so above.

In the spiritual world everything is in motion and transition, and is in continuous development.

According to Rudolf Steiner in his course on light[1], even time and space are based on movement.

Also, nothing repeats itself, a specific experience can never be experienced twice.

All development in the spirit is based on movement, transition, change, transformation and translocation.

In obtaining clairvoyance we have also to move in the spiritual world and translocate something or make some change in the established order of our soul properties, our spiritual make-up.

To treat a patient, we have to change something, make something move. We have to transform or to translocate.

Quite early in my career as a veterinarian I made some astonishing observations.

These observations were based on the foundation of finding the true cause of the disease and not by focusing on the symptoms.

---

[1] See GA 320, a series of 11 lectures given in Stuttgart for teachers in the Walldorf-school. The series started 23rd of December 1919, ending on the 3rd of January 1920.

To do this I had to learn methods to develop a more sensitive energetic observation of the body than usually are used within ordinary veterinary or human medicine.

For the most part I used (and still use) pulse-diagnosis, but also incorporated a certain clairvoyance and general/special sensitivity.

My observations were (described in 8 points):

1. In treating animals, I found that the deeper cause of the disease *in the animals* **almost always** was the same as the deeper cause in the owner.
2. In treating humans, I found that the deeper cause of the symptoms **usually** was the same in the children as in the dominating parent.
3. In treating humans, I found that the deeper cause of the symptoms **often** was the same as in the spouse, especially if the spouse was the dominating partner.
4. I found that in treating the alpha-human (the origin of the deeper cause of the disease) in a **transformative** way, a healing process was induced in the **whole** family and farm-animals.
5. I found that the use of 5-elemenal thinking[2] furthers 'translocation' of the deeper cause, while using systems based on 7- or 12-element thinking[3] furthers a 'transformation'. A 6-element[4] thinking furthers a 'suppression' of the symptoms.

---

[2] Most of the acupuncture philosophy and practice is based on the 5-element theory and the conception of Yin/Yang, and as I often use acupuncture in my treatment I had the ability to observe these connections.

[3] The so called 5-elements can be ordered differently and arranged according to the 7 planets and also to the 12 zodiacal signs. This view will as such then correlate more with anthroposophy than Chinese philosophy and thinking.

[4] As the 5-element thinking of the Chinese can be transformed or adjusted to both a 7-elemet and a 12-element thinking, it can also be adopted to a 6-element thinking.

a. 5-elemental thinking as a representative for the eastern way of thinking (Chinese thinking, Buddhism, Taoism, Hinduism).
b. 6-elemental thinking as a representative for the middle-east way of thinking (Islamic, Jewish).
c. 7- or 12-element thinking as a representative for the European-western way of thinking (Christian, Anthroposophic).

6. When I regularly monitored the health of animals, especially horses, and they were sold to another person, the deepest cause of their symptoms changed from being like the old alfa-owner to be like the new alfa-owner as soon as the animal accepted the new owner as his alfa-'master'. Also when a young woman who was living with her dominant mother, and thus showed the same 'deficiency' as the mother, married a dominant man, she changed the 'deeper cause (in several of my books also called the 'deficient' organ) in three years.

7. The described 'deeper cause' of the disease showed different symptoms, in relation to where in the body this deeper cause found its expression. A kidney weakness in the human remained a kidney weakness in the animal, but it expressed itself very differently, depending on where in the body 'it' (the kidney weakness) found a 'home', found a 'hold' (see table next page).

For example:

Symptoms that may arise from a poor blood circulation (the deficient process) are very variable. Symptoms differ according to the time of the year, the age and the species or breed of the animal or human patient.

Poor blood circulation (in acupuncture called TH, Trippel Heather) manifests differently with different species, gender and ages:

Species, gender and age	Poor blood circulation manifests as
Children	Otitis media
Young girls and boys	Eczema
Puberty girls	Menstrual problems, painful
Puberty boys	Acne
Older women, menopausal women	"Heat" Syndromes (internal heat after menstruation); hot flushes (vasomotor disorders)
Grown up men	Back pain
Puppies	Red skin infections around the nose
Young dogs	Furunculosis, skin infections of the paws
Trotters	Fetlock, or navicular disorders, especially on the right forelimb
Cows	Mastitis

8. I found that if there were no 'homes' or 'places of hold' in the beta-human or child or animal, the transferred disease-cause or weakness was not allowed to come to expression, but remained dormant (sub-clinical).

As we will see later in this book, and as it is described in several of my other books, especially *"Demons and Healing"* and *"Experiences from the Threshold"*[5], the reason for all these observations, and also the only logical explanation, is that diseases are expressions of spiritual beings, called distorted (changed) elemental beings or 'demons' (pathological elemental beings). These beings are able to travel from a human being to an animal, between humans and also between animals.

In treatment the easiest wat to 'heal' a person is to just translocate the problem, the demon. It is more difficult to transform the demon. That is why several schools, especially in China, have this

---

[5] Both published on 'Temple Lodge', 2018 and 2019.

knowledge, and try to translocate the demons into plants or semiprecious stones[6].

Most European schools of acupuncture also have this knowledge, but are not consciously aware of it, as they actually teach their students how to avoid a translocation to themselves, but do not consider that 'the disease' can translocate to others.

With this understanding and insight, I will summarize the most important concepts that will be the foundation of all the further understandings in this book:

- All physical phenomena and beings have a spiritual foundation, a spiritual reality.
- In the spiritual world all entities or part of an entity can translocate and transform, both the beneficial and the adversary ones.
  - When a beneficial entity or part translocate or transform our level of consciousness is changed.
  - When a malignant or adversarial entity or part of this entity translocate or transform in a negative way, disease is created, aggravated or translocated.
- All diseases or symptoms in both humans, animals and plants are physical expressions of the presence of non-beneficial spiritual entities.
- These spiritual, non-beneficial entities might be toxic plant spirits, bacterial spirits, viral spirits, old Karmic spirits or other forms of demonic spirits.
- All such pathological spirits seek a home or living place in the body, an empty or weak void to slip into.
- All adversarial spirits are of three different kinds, sometimes operating on their own, sometimes operating together, as in cancer as we later will see.

---

[6] Personal communication from the Chinese translator of "Demons and Healing" (ongoing translation).

The three kinds are:
- ○ Ahrimanic spirits.
- ○ Luciferic spirits.
- ○ Azuric spirits.
- All the different symptoms in both humans and animals come from one of these three spiritual 'demons' entering through one of the 12 sense-openings and taking possession of one of 12 possible voids (the 12 main organs) in the body.
- The demons may enter via the 12 different sensory organs of the body, each belonging to one zodiacal energy stream.
- These 36 different possibilities can give rise to a thousand symptoms in the different species and different individual humans.
- All these different symptoms can be treated by treating the fundamental cause, the original 'demon', usually coming from the dominant alfa-human.
- All internal diseases in animals come from humans.
- In treatment or therapy all diseases can either be **translocated** or **transformed** (not the symptoms, but the causative 'demon').
- To understand the mechanism of such translocation we need to understand the:
  - ○ Development and spiritual construction of the entire cosmos.
  - ○ Development and spiritual construction of man.
  - ○ Development and spiritual construction of animals.
  - ○ The reality and substance of the translocated disease.
- To be able to diagnose the diseases spiritually we have to enter the spiritual world through our **feeling** and also develop some kind of 'monitoring' of these pathological entities, as for example through the use of pulse diagnosis.
- To be able to treat the diseases spiritually we have to enter the spiritual world through our **willing** and also develop some kind of method to 'influence' these pathological

entities inside the patient's body, for example through herbs, acupuncture, homeopathy or osteopathy.
- The effect of both diagnosis and treatment is highly dependent on the insights and knowledge of the therapist.
- Christ is the main and fundamental transforming force.

In all these explanations I will describe the spiritual foundation as given by **Rudolf Steiner**, and also in certain aspects by **Edgar Cayce** and **Peter Deunov (Beinsa Douno)**.

Rudolf Steiner regarding the concept of shared diseases.
Using the words of the Biblical Gospel according to Luke, on September 24th, 1909, Rudolf Steiner lectured on the importance of the concept of shared demonic pathology among all beings and its treatment with Christ Consciousness.

"At the time of Christ's appearance on the Earth there were many human beings in His environment in whom sins and transgressions — especially defects of character deriving from former bad traits — were expressing themselves in disease. The sin that is actually seated in the astral body and manifests as illness, is called 'possession' in the Gospel of St. Luke. It is the condition that sets in when a man attracts alien spirits into his astral body and when his better qualities fail to give him mastery over his whole nature. In human beings in whom the old state of separation between the etheric and physical bodies still persisted, the effects of evil qualities and attributes expressed themselves conspicuously at that time in forms of illness manifesting as 'possession'. The Gospel of St. Luke tells how such people were healed through the mere proximity and the words of the individuality of Christ Jesus and how the evil power working in them was expelled. This is a prefigurement of conditions at the end of Earth evolution, when man's good qualities will exercise a healing influence upon all his other traits."

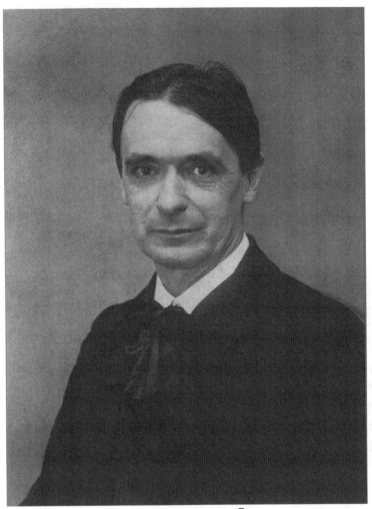

Rudolf Steiner[7]

---

[7] **Rudolf Joseph Lorenz Steiner** (25. February 1861 – 30 March 1925) was an Austrian philosopher, author, social reformer, architect and esoterist. Steiner gained initial recognition at the end of the nineteenth century as a literary critic and published philosophical works including *"The Philosophy of Freedom"*. At the beginning of the twentieth century, he founded an esoteric Spiritual movement, Anthroposophy, with roots in German idealist philosophy and theosophy. Other influences include Goethean science and Rosecrucianism. In the first, more

philosophically oriented phase of this movement, Steiner attempted to find a synthesis between science and Spirituality. His philosophical work from these years, which he termed Spiritual science, sought to apply the clarity of thinking characteristic of western philosophy to Spiritual questions differentiating this approach from what he considered to be vague approaches to mysticism. In the second phase, beginning around 1907, he began working collaboratively in a variety of artistic media, including drama, the movement arts (developing a new artistic form, eurythmy) and architecture, culminating in the building of the Goetheanum, a cultural center to house all the activities of Anthroposophy. In the third phase of his work, beginning after world war I, Steiner worked to establish various practical endeavors, including Waldorf education, biodynamic agriculture, and anthroposophical medicine. Steiner advocated a form of ethical individualism, to which he later brought a more explicitly Spiritual approach. He based his epistemology on Johann Wolfgang von Goethe's worldview, in which "Thinking ... is no more and no less an organ of perception than the eye or ear. Just as the eye perceives colors and the ear sounds, so thinking perceives ideas." A consistent thread that runs from his earliest philosophical phase through his later Spiritual orientation is the goal of Demonstrating that there are no essential limits to human knowledge. In 1899 Steiner experienced what he described as a life-transforming inner encounter with the being of Christ; previously he had little or no relation to Christianity in any form. Then and thereafter, his relationship to Christianity remained entirely founded upon personal experience, and was thus both non-denominational and strikingly different from conventional religious forms. Steiner was then 38 years of age, and the experience of meeting the Christ occurred after a tremendous inner struggle. To use Steiner's own words, the "experience culminated in my standing in the Spiritual presence of the mystery of Golgotha in a most profound and solemn festival of knowledge."

All of my earlier books are each about a specific part of the spiritual world and the experiences I have had in that part.

- *Poplar* is about the spiritual experiences I had in nature, especially with trees, leading back to early childhood.
- *7-fold Way to Therapy* is about the spiritual experiences I had in developing my therapeutic methods, especially relating to the so-called "First Class" of Rudolf Steiner (1924).
- *The Forgotten Mysteries of Atlantis* is about the spiritual experiences I had in understanding my personal karma, especially in relation to my work.
- *Alternative Veterinary Medicine* is about the spiritual experiences I had as a veterinarian, in trying to find my way from the materialistic medicine of today towards a more spiritual practice.
- *Demons and Healing* is about the spiritual experiences I had in meeting the demonic entities causing disease and creating misfortune.
- *Spiritual Medicine* is about the spiritual experiences I had resulting in the later development of my therapeutic methods, especially in the finding of the Christ force that resides in the middle of "everything", and also in understanding the huge danger and illusionary scam that 5 element acupuncture (Traditional Chinese Medicine (TCM)) has led us into.
- *Experiences from the Threshold* is about the experiences I have had in passing the threshold.

These books are all about one thing: to understand man, nature, plants, animals and medicine from a spiritual world view. By spiritual world view I mean a world view based on the existence of "spirits".

Spirits are "behind" and are fundamental to all material existence, to plants, animals and man, yes, to the whole earth.

The spiritual world is also 'behind' all kind of diseases, how they are created and how they spread.

To be able to write the books referred to here, I had first to cross the 'Threshold' to the spiritual world. The techniques I have used to do so I call "Translocation" of spiritual parts of my total spiritual composition.
To write the medical books and practice my way of medicine I have to understand and being able to either Translocate or Transform the spiritual entities causing disease, the demonic forces.

- *'Translocation' as the cause of disease and of spiritual movability and initiation.*
- *'Transformation' as the cause of healing and spiritual development.*

In my book **"Spiritual Medicine"**, I explain the spiritual foundations of my therapeutic methods, especially related to the Christ force. To use this Christ-force, I have to 'transform' and not 'translocate' the adversarial forces causing disease and hindering Christ, namely the ahrimanic-, azuric- and the luciferic forces.

All internal diseases are caused by demons, distorted elemental beings, created by our wrong thoughts, egoistic feelings and evil actions.

The implications of translocation within human and veterinary medicine.

The void into which alien entities may enter.

The upsetting claim that all diseases in both man and women, in their children and in their animals have their origin in the human entity needs some explanation.

All diseases are translocated from the 'strongest' (alpha-being) human being to the animal.

Such translocation can also happen between adults and children, and also between adults themselves. It then usually is translocated from a stronger human being to a weaker one.

This is why diseases almost never translocate from animals to humans, although this might happen. Likewise, with weaker humans and children, they are usually the suffering target of such translocation.

We have then to understand:

- *what is translocated?*
- *how can such translocated 'items' cause disease?*

So, what is this "something", inhabiting the body, that can translocate?!

The first time I saw this 'something' was in Bodø in 1980, when I was a veterinarian in this area of Northern Norway. This day my wife (at that time) had a visit from a friend. When I came into the room I *saw* a "structure" half way out of her friends left scull, half way within the head. It was like a spiral, similar to a curled snake or a skein of wool. She told me that she was suffering from a painful migraine. I went towards this woman, and took hold of the energetic "structure" with my hand. I pulled the "structure" half way out, and the woman said that the pain diminished, almost disappeared. Then I let go of the "structure", and it slipped immediately back into the head of the woman. *"Auuuu"* she said, *"now the pain has come back"*!

Again, I grabbed hold of the "structure" and pulled it all the way out. The migraine totally disappeared. I was very careful with what I did to the "structure" that I held in my hand. I went to the open window, and threw the "structure" out.

It did not return.

In the following years, in fact until today, I have asked myself again and again:

- ***What was that structure, from where had it come and where did it go after I threw it out of the window?***
- ***Did it come back?***
- ***Did it go to someone else?***

These questions became very important for me. The answers to these questions are essential to:

Understanding the existence of such pathological structures (later in this book called demons), how they are translocated and their part in disease, especially the human-animal pathological connection.

Often when I treated diseases with homeopathy or acupuncture, which I have used much in my practice on animals and their owners, the symptoms often moved around in the body. Over 3-4 months of repeated treatment a migraine could move down into the hand and stay as a pain in the little finger for some time before it vanished in the thin air. As a medically trained person I know that migraine is caused by a pulsating artery that affects a nerve in the head, so this moving around appeared quite strange to me, quite unexplainable.

I then had to pose the very important question to myself:

"What is it that travels from the brain into the little finger and after a while disappears?"

Then I began to see and understand more and more what the reality behind the "travelling structures" of diseases was.

They are structures that have their own life, which can travel in the body from top to bottom. They can also jump over to another person, or to an animal. Not only CAN they do this, this jumping and travelling and changing is a fundamental property of these demons.

They are structures that are alive. Ordinary treatment with physiotherapy, osteopathy, acupuncture, painkillers and other allopathic medicines usually only move these structures to other places in the body or to other individuals.

In discussing this phenomenon with colleges, both acupuncturists, zone-therapists and even Chi-Gong-therapists, they are all aware of the danger that such 'entities' shall 'jump over' to themselves, and they are very careful to prevent this from happening. To prevent this is actually a part of their education.

Very few have given the thought, that such 'pathological entities' can jump over to others, to the wife or neighbor when they come home, to the horse when they go to the stable or to their children, a proper and serious consideration.

In my practice, as well in the practices of all my colleges, I became painfully aware that we all just translocate the noxious structures called 'demons', the symptoms, and for this we receive money!

If one reviews the literature of various alternative medical systems, there are revelations that show this translocation phenomena was already being observed by some of the great physicians of homeopathy, such as Dr. Constantine Hering[8], the author of Hering's Laws of Cure.[9]

---

[8] Dr. Constantine Hering M.D. (1800-1880). Dr. Hering is aptly called the "Father of Homoeopathy" in America. Originally a skeptic of homeopathy, he was convinced of its efficacy after an objective study of its principles. He went on to expound upon the Laws of cure.

[9] Hering's Law of Cure. This law states:
- Cure occurs from above and downwards. It progresses from the head towards the lower trunk, that is to say the head symptoms clear first. With regard to the extremities, cure spreads from shoulder to fingers, or hip to toes.
- Cure occurs from within outwards and progresses from more important organs (e.g. liver, endocrine system) to less important organs (e.g. joints). That is to say, the function of vital organs is restored before those less important to life. The end result of this externalization of disease is often the production of "treatment cutaneous rash".
- Symptoms appear in reverse chronological order. More recent symptoms and pathology will clear before old, the disease "backtracks" so to speak.

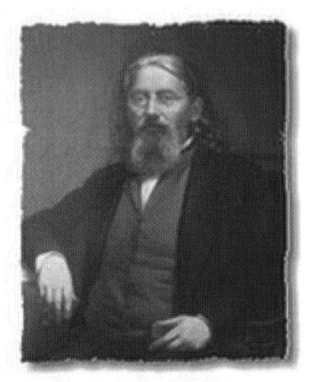

Constantine Hering
1800 - 1880

The name "demon" calls forth disbelief in many readers. I could have called the described these demonic entities as *"pathological or noxious structures of either Yin or Yang quality with their own life"*, but this would not be honest.

I prefer to call them by their old name, demons.

- The *"pathological or noxious structure of Yin quality with its own life"* I call an ahrimanic demon.
- The *"pathological or noxious structure of Yang quality with its own life"* I call a luciferic demon[10].

When we treat, either with homeopathy, acupuncture or herbs, there are two possible outcomes from a seemingly successful treatment;

- the pathological structure is dissolved, transformed,
- or it is translocated.

If we treat the symptoms (which we may call the excess), even if we treat the cause (which we may call the deficiency), the pathological structure may just be transposed, translocated. We think then that the disease is healed, but it is just hidden, symptomatically changed, moved or translocated to another being.

For a long time, I have observed this occurrence, both for me and for my colleges. I would say that it happens in:

- 100 % of all allopathic (school medicine) treatments and in
- 90% of all alternative treatments when the excess is addressed, that is the area of pain or symptoms. It happens in
- 10% when the deficiency is addressed, and mostly when treatment according to the:
  - 5-elements is used. It rarely happens when a treatment according to:

---

[10] When my book «Demons – Healing» published by «Temple Lodge» (Forest Row, England), was translated into Chinese, the translator contacted me, telling me this knowledge is actually still valid in China. Many acupuncturists know of the phenomenon of translocation, and some try to make the demon go into plants or stones. She further told that the secrets of the 6-, 7- and 12-elements was partly hidden, partly unknown in China.

o   7- or 12-elements is used.
- Seldom when the 90^0 method is used (see
- Sometimes when the star-method is used
o   Almost never when the middle-point is addressed)[11]

The most important question for me in these latter years has been how to dissolve or transform the disease-causing elementals called 'demons', and not just translocate them to others.

This described translocation gives the foundation of the observed pathological connection between all living entities.

There is a strong energetic connection between all levels of creation, and we are all connected energetically through the existence of the elementals[12], both the benign beings and the malign beings, the so-called demons.

There are 3 types of demons.
In the spiritual world on the other side of the threshold, there are many kinds of entities, just as in the physical world. Here in the

---

[11] There are many more details about this in my book «Spiritual Medicine».

[12] There are many stories and insights from old times and old religions where disease and ailments are looked upon as separate and individualized entities, or energetically self-conscious structures, described as elementals, spirits, demons or devas. Many of us have experienced that if we are too open in the moment of acupuncture treatment, the energetic pathological structure may jump over and attack us, inflict us with the disease itself. We have also seen that such pathological structures may inflict, influence or create disease in creatures connected to the patient. We are all interwoven in an enormous web of energy, a web that connects all living entities in the world, maybe even the whole cosmos. This web is to be seen just on the other side of the threshold to the Spiritual world. It is called by many names: the Akashic record, Karma or the Matrix. This web is made of energy, but not just lifeless aimless energy. It is made up of elementals, living etheric beings, created by human minds, our thoughts, feelings and actions. This web is also part of our diseases, and is influenced when we treat energetically.

physical world, we may meet innumerable types of beings, some are beneficial to us, some are indifferent and some are dangerous. In the spiritual world it is just as in the physical world, and those beings or entities that are dangerous to us we call "adversaries".

There are many different types of these adversaries, but to make it easier to define them we may divide them into three groups:

- the ahrimanic beings, "demons or ahrimanic demons", which are ahrimanic adversarial entities in the etheric realm, which want us to be more materialistic and deny the spiritual world.
- the luciferic beings, "specters or luciferic demons", which are luciferic adversarial entities in the astral realm, which want us to lose ourselves in our own subjective experiences of the spiritual world.
- the azuric beings, "phantoms or azuric demons", which are azuric adversarial entities in both the physical and spiritual realms, attacking the physical body as well as the "I" or "I organization", who want us to lose our "I", or make the "I" egoistic and unsuitable for the spiritual world.

I mentioned earlier that if we are not conscious inside our separated soul parts with our awakened "I", then alien and malignant forces have the possibility of entering our being. A meeting with these powers, internal or external, seems to be inevitable when working with crossing the threshold and passing into the spiritual world.

All diseases have their origin in the spiritual world, caused by the presence of demonic structures.

How are Demons created?
On what do they "feed"?
Earth-radiation and Karma.

How are Demons created?

I have come to understand that they are all created by evil or egoistic deeds of humans, and feed on the upward streaming forces of the deeper layers of the earth. If the human being that created the elemental demon is dead, a grid-line in the earth, which we today call 'earth-radiation' still remains as a trace or mark of the deed. In the period when the originator of the grid-line has entered the spiritual world, i.e. is dead, the grid-line is left alone here in the physical world. Here it may cause disease or discomfort in other humans or animals that happen to sleep or live where the lines are. In a later life, when the originator of the line is reincarnated, the spirit of this reincarnated human is drawn to the site where 'the line' awaits. When he or she then comes again to the area of past sin, the past misdeed, the grid-lines (demons) attach to the human who then consciously or unconsciously remembers these past actions. It is known within criminology that the perpetrator always returns to the site of the crime.

The earth-radiation lines are really elementals. If they are created by benevolent deeds they are just called 'elementals'. If they are created by malevolent deeds they are called demonic elementals or demons, and they are disease creating, connected to our Karma. If the originator is in the otherworld, the demons may haunt other people whilst they wait for their "makers" to be re-born.

These lines or grids contain the whole history of our lives, and as such they may be called *"The Akasha Chronicle"*[13]. Karma and the

---

[13] **Akasha** (Sanskrit ākāśa आकाश) is a term for "æther" in traditional Indian cosmology. The term has also been adopted in western occultism and

Akashic Chronicle are interwoven in this grid, and are two parts or realities of the earth radiation.

It must be understood the whole world is full of these Demons, Demonic Grids fed by the upward streaming of ahrimanic forces from the depths.

They are of many kinds and appearances.

Some are made by greed, others from anger, through murder, violence, jealousy and from pain or sorrow.

Demons will also be created through deeds of violence towards nature.

If we cut down a tree, if we kill weeds or insects by the help of chemicals (Roundup), if we slaughter a healthy cow or horse, if we cut down whole areas of forest with huge machines, strong disharmonic demons will be created that later can translocate to humans and further to animals.

Spiritualism in the late 19th century. The Sanskrit word is derived from a root kāś meaning "to be visible". It appears as a masculine noun in Vedic Sanskrit with a generic meaning of "open space, vacuity". In Classical Sanskrit, the noun acquires the neuter gender and may express the concept of "sky; atmosphere" (Manusmrti, Shatapathabrahmana). In classical Vedantic Hindu philosophy, the word acquires its technical meaning of "an ethereal fluid imagined as pervading the cosmos". In many modern Indo-Aryan languages, the corresponding word (often rendered Akash) retains a generic meaning of "sky". The Western religious philosophy called Theosophy has popularized the word Akasha as an adjective, through the use of the term "Akashic records" or "Akashic library", referring to an ethereal compendium of all knowledge and history. **Scott Cunningham** (1995) uses the term Akasha to refer to "the Spiritual force that Earth, Air, Fire, and Water descend from". **Ervin László** in Science and the Akashic Field: An Integral Theory of Everything (2004), based on ideas by **Rudolf Steiner**, posits "a field of information" as the substance of the cosmos, which he calls "Akashic field".

Demons can be divided in two groups according to when and how they were created:

1. Demons created by human actions.
2. Demons existing from earlier cosmic development.

I find it extremely difficult to make a differentiation between these two groups, as both groups appear quite equal. However, I know from my work that they are different.

Demons are always involved in the development of disease, occurring in animals and in man.

Concerning diseases in humans relating to both the body and the soul, the most significant demons are those we have created ourselves through our actions, thoughts and feelings. They may be called our "karmic" demons, or the karmic 'doppelgänger'.

Example:

I was visiting a friend of mine. He was often thrown into severe depressions, and could not work for weeks or months. He had no idea from where these depressions came. At the time I was visiting him he was in a better period. I sat at the table and he went to the kitchen to make me a coffee, an espresso. As he was doing this a huge, dark shadow slowly engulfed him, and he sank into a dark mood. This dark mood that descended upon him was the cause of his repeated depressions. I tried to ask the Demon from whence it came, but it would not answer. I further asked the entity how old it was, and finally it responded that it had been created by a dark action committed by my friends´ grandfather. The action had to do with an act of low morality.

The next step would be to find out what this was, and then ask for forgiveness. If this is properly performed, the Demon will disperse and vanish, having been freed and transformed. We must not just push the Demon away. *It wants to be transformed*.

Demons and "earth-radiation".

The so-called "earth-radiation" has two aspects:

- The semi-physical expression of the created demons
- The upstreaming forces of evil beings from early history of the world, residing in the deeper layers of the world.

This etheric forces from the depths of the earth are very central in understanding the nature of demons, ahrimanic beings and disease.

My development in seeing and understanding earth-radiation is much the same as my path in seeing and understanding pathologic demons.

I understood from early on that they belong together, that they are one and the same.

Since 1972 I have been investigating the so-called *"leylines"* and earth grids called *"earth-radiation"*, especially since from 2004 when I began to **see** this matrix of energy[14]. This energy is *spiritual energy* as no one has as yet been able to prove the existence of it with electric instruments or other kinds of devices. It can only be detected by living beings.

I am aware that there is also a huge grid of electromagnetic energy that causes disease in living beings. This is especially noticeable in connection with emissions from high-voltage installations and cell phones. This is something I will come back to later in chapter 5, but

---

[14] Described in my book "Holistic Veterinary Medicine" published on Amazon. It can also be obtained in Norwegian, Swedish, Spanish, German and Italian. Also described in my book "Poplar", published on Amazon, which can also be obtained in Norwegian (Poppel) and German (Pappel).

here I will write about the spiritual energetic grid that has a spiritual origin.

The *spiritual energy* on which the demons are feeding is an emanation from the demonic layers of the earth itself. At the same time it is also the expression of the ahrimanic entities created by human misdeeds throughout all times. This "spiritual substance" is thus both the demonic entities themselves and a kind of fuel or food for the ahrimanic entities.

Such emanations fuel the karmic demons and cause disease, especially if one sleeps over this radiation or is connected to it.

This matrix or grid of earth-radiation is changeable, **it is alive and has its own intent**.

The next level of my observations was as follows: I discovered that the lines of earth-radiation not only changed, but moved several meters by themselves, especially if someone tried to alter, disperse or stop them.

Then I made the astonishing observation that they could also **be moved by my own will and intent**.

I started to demonstrate this possibility to dowsers. During a dowsing congress I moved a "lay-line" through the room so fast that many of the participants felt it like a soft wind that swept through the room.

I carry out this moving of earth-radiation according to the following method; first I have to "see" the energetic lines.[15] After seeing the

---

[15] **Earth-Radiation** is "seen" (at least I see it this way) as snakes traversing the room, or the forest. Black and shiny, going from left to right or from right to left. One direction goes from the past to the future, and the other direction goes from the future to the past. At a certain level this energy has the shape of a snake, on a higher level it has the shape of a Demon. Before 2014 I saw the

energy (the 'snakes') I fixate it with my Will power, just as we might fixate a naughty child when we require its attention or when we want the child to acts as we wish. Then I move the 'snake' by "Willpower and Intent" to another place. This technique is much the same as I use to move the "northern lights" as described in chapter 5.

They follow my "command" and move.

In the Old Norse book *"Edda"*[16] a similar structure or phenomenon as the 'earth-radiation' and deep upstreaming forces of the earth is described, relating to the *"Nornes"*[17]. The Old Vikings *"saw"* that when a child was born, a *"web"* was waiting for it. Three women were waiting to connect the child to this web, which was the karma of this newborn being. The names of the three women were past, present and future (Vilje, Ve and Verdande). The "Nornes" also had scissors to cut the thread when the task of this life was fulfilled. This is for me an accurate description of the karmic web, the cause of its existence and how it is created.

I observe this karmic web in connection with all human beings.

Demons in the shape of snakes, and mainly as "earth-radiation". Lately I can see them as Demons, clinging to humans, causing diseases and pain, depressions or anger. Even Death can be seen in this way.

[16] The term **"Edda"** (/ˈɛdə/; Old Norse Edda, plural Eddur) applies to the Old Norse Edda and has been adapted to fit the collection of poems known as the Poetic Edda which lacks an original title. Both works were written down in Iceland during the 13th century, although they contain material from earlier traditional sources, relating back to the Viking Age. These books are the main sources of medieval skaldic tradition in Icelandic and Norse mythology.

[17] The **Norns** (Old Norse: norn, plural: nornir) in Norse mythology are female beings who rule the destiny of gods and men. They roughly correspond to other controllers of humans' destiny, the Fates, elsewhere in European mythology. According to Snorri Sturluson's interpretation of the Völuspá, the three most important norns, Urðr (Wyrd), Verðandi and Skuld, come out from a hall standing at the Well of Urðr (well of fate, KARMA).

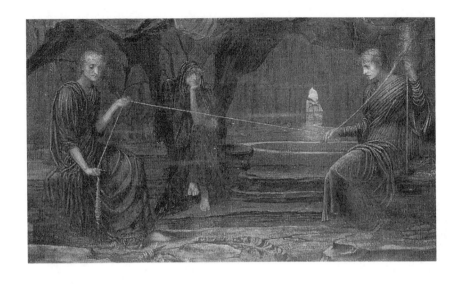

The three Nornes

When I stared to understand this, I clearly saw the connections between "Earth-Radiation" and humans. I saw how the actions of man created or attracted (translocation) the snakes/demons, and how these demons created diseases and disasters in man.

Such demons may also create disease in people who live close by or are attached to those who carry the demons (translocation).

It has been observed throughout time that living or sleeping on "earth-radiation" may cause disease, and also that it is impossible to free yourself from these demons, unless you know how.

The void.

When an elemental spirit, a demon or any other benign or malign spirit enters you, influences you or actually possesses you, there must be an empty room available, some weakness or a void into where it is possible to in-dwell.

This is of utmost importance to know relating to:

- Spiritual possessions.
- Use of alcohol or drugs.
- Development of diseases.
- Hypersensitivity.
- Exposure to electro-magnetic radiation.
- Openness to Ahriman and Lucifer.

In the beginning of man's evolution, we ourselves used this method or possibility of entering or possessing other beings, entering into the void of their spiritual construction.

According to **Edgar Cayce** when the first 'group' of human souls entered the earth sphere in the Lemurian times, they entered into or actually possessed animal forms, to experience the pleasures of the earthly existence (in 'Genesis' they were called the sons or daughters of **man**). But alas, they were trapped in these forms, not able to reenter the spiritual world.

The next group of souls entering the earthly realm was the 'rescue party' who came to help the trapped sons of man back to God, incarnating in human forms, which later were developed to reach the perfection of life that can house a conscious "I". This second group (in 'Genesis' they were called the sons or daughters of **God**) came to help or rescue the first group and free them from the material prison they had put themselves in. This second group was also trapped deeply into materialism due to the cunny plans of the devil, and in the end Christ himself had to come to rescue them all.

According to **Rudolf Steiner** the animal forms were created as side-products to the human development, but still some of the immature human souls incarnated too soon and gave life to apes and higher animals, who must be considered as our brothers and sisters and need our help and salvation.

A healthy human being fills out his or her physical body entirely with the etheric and astral sheets. But, there are very few healthy humans, we are all weakened somewhat and somewhere, depending on our individual lives, individual karma and individual beliefs.

It is important to understand that how we eat, how we think or act, how our moral behavior influences out lives make certain weaknesses in our spiritual/physical make-up. Such weaknesses create portals through which alien spirits or spiritual influences may enter.

If we for example have no consciousness about our food and eat fast food every day such as is found at McDonalds, then, after a few weeks or months, our liver will be weakened in its etheric make-up so much that it will be open for an alien invasion or the creation of adversary entities. An ahrimanic spirit can develop from our own etheric forces or an already created ahrimanic demon can enter. This creates a *'deficient'* disease, as the symptoms then always show a lessening of activity. This ahrimanic elemental demonic entity invites or creates a luciferic demon, and this demon shows considerably more clear symptoms than the ahrimanic one, and is thus called an *'excessive'* disease. Therefore, most diseases are a cooperation between the ahrimanic and the luciferic demons, the luciferic dwelling cranial (towards the head) and the ahrimanic dwelling distal (towards the feet). Between these two we find the middle-point, or the area I call the 'Christ-point'. If we strengthen this area, the two adversarial forces will be transformed and weakened.

Other causes for opening for an invasion of adversarial forces may be the use of alcohol and drugs.

If for example there is too big an opening in the defensive power of the body due to a weakening of the etheric or astral strength, certain portals may be created, and through such portals alien entities or influences may enter, and the result is often seen as hypersensitivity and allergy.

The hypersensitivity of electromagnetic radiation (EMR) will be dealt with in chapter 6.

There are to my knowledge in principle four ways to help or treat such an influx of entities or unwanted spirituality due to having a too wide opening of portals or weakening of the protective force of the etheric or astral sheet.

1. **Translocate** the spirits out (as in exorcism).
2. Make room for the Christ force in the middle to **transform** the unwanted luciferic or ahrimanic spirits.
3. **Close the 'door'** that allows the spirits in.
4. **Fill the void** by changing the detrimental way of living.

Understanding and mastering the mechanism of translocation and transformation, both in humans and in the animal kingdom.

To understand the mechanism involved in the translocation of diseases from man to animals, we first have to describe the spiritual development and composition of:

- the **cosmos**, as an expression of both the human and the animal development.
- the development of **man**.
- the development of **animals**.
- the common evolution of **both man and animals**.

Then we will understand how translocations can occur.

The development of our common cosmos.

Steiner explained that mankind as well as Earth have, so far, passed through three major stages which he called **"Old Saturn," "Old Sun"**, and **"Old Moon"**. We are currently now in the phase of the Earth that we now inhabit (**Present Earth**). He also claimed that the present planets of the solar system are evolutionary descendants of their namesakes. For example, the planet Saturn as we see it now, is a remnant of the planetary condition called 'Old Saturn'. In a way, the planets of Anthroposophy actually represent a time line of our evolution towards our highest I.

The future incarnations of both our solar system, our spirituality and our karmic path are **"future Jupiter", "future Venus"** and **"future Vulcan"**.[18]

---

[18] **Future Jupiter:** After the dissolution of Earth, the entire universe will reincarnate as the Jupiter phase, the 5th planetary phase, as a mirror image of 'Old Moon'. The concept of imagination will at this time be perfected and its inhabitants will be formed out of human will through the pineal gland.

The development of man.

In 1907 Rudolf Steiner wrote:

We shall most easily understand the progress of humanity through the three incarnations, Saturn, Sun, and Moon, preceding the Earth, if we add a further survey of man in sleep, in dream. When man is asleep the seer beholds the astral body with the ego enveloped in it as though floating over the physical body. The astral body is then outside the physical and etheric bodies, but remains connected with them. It sends threads, as it were, or rather currents into the universal cosmic body, and seems partly embedded in it. Thus, in the sleeping man we have the physical, the etheric and the astral body, and this last sends out tentacles towards the great astral universe. If we picture this condition as an enduring one, if here on the physical plane there were only human beings who had the physical body interpenetrated with the etheric body, while above hovered over them an astral soul with the ego, then we should have the condition in which mankind existed on the Moon. Except that on the Moon the astral body was not strongly separated from the physical body; it sank down into the physical body just as strongly as it expanded into the cosmos. But if you picture a state of sleep where no dream ever comes then you have the

---

Future Venus represents the 6th planetary phase as a mirror image of the 'Old Sun'. When mankind ascends to this level of his evolution, he will perfect the stage of inspiration. In addition, our etheric sheath will develop complete consciousness. We will have conscious sleep and see the spirit world. In fact, those who have become initiated can exist in this future now.

Future Vulcan: This planetary phase, the 7th, represents the final planetary condition as the mirror image of 'Old Saturn'. Only the most highly evolved humans will progress to this phase. It is at this time that we perfect the stage of intuition. In reaching Vulcan, we will recapitulate all the stages of our evolution. At this point mankind will be completely spiritualized, that is living entirely in the spirit without any physical body.

condition in which humanity existed on the Sun. And if you now imagine that the human being has died, that even his etheric body is outside him, united to the astral body and ego, but yet that the link is not quite dissolved, so that what is outside, embedded in the whole surrounding cosmos, sends down its rays and works upon the physical substance — you then have the condition in which mankind existed on Saturn (Steiner GA 99, 1907).

Human beings were actually already in existence on Saturn but in a dull, dull consciousness. These souls in an active and mobile state had the task of maintaining something that belonged to them 'down below'. They worked from above on their physical body, like a snail fashioning its shell; they acted from outside, just like an instrument, on the bodily organs. We will describe the appearance of that on which the souls above were working; we must give some little description of this physical Saturn, of Saturn in general.

When each planet has completed its evolution and becomes spiritual again, it is, so to speak, no longer in existence. It passes over into a condition of sleep (Pralaya) in order to come forth once more.

This development has passed through the planetary stages of Saturn, Sun and Moon, is (as described above) at the present Earth-stage, and in the coming epochs will pass through future Jupiter, future Venus and culminating in the Vulcan-development.

- **Saturn-evolution**: consisted of a development in pure warmth, and the differences between the epochs were not so distinct as is here now on the Earth, the Saturn evolution also consisted of the 7x7x7 epochs.

Following the 'Saturn-incarnation' the 'Earth´s' next incarnation was the 'Sun'.

- **Sun-evolution**: this was a mix of all that is on the present sun, moon and earth, blended together with all the terrestrial and spiritual beings alive in our solar system today. The Sun evolution was distinguished by the fact that the etheric body then drew into the physical body which had already been prepared on Saturn. The Sun had a denser substantiality than Saturn, and can be likened with the density of our present air. The human physical substance, which was formed on Saturn from pure warmth, was interpenetrated on the Sun by the etheric body. Our bodies thus became bodies of air and light, adding to the warmth body developed on Saturn. 'We' worked (actually it was the higher beings that were the ones that worked) down into the physical and etheric bodies, just as today in sleep when our astral body is outside, and works upon the physical and the etheric body. At that time, we were forming the first rudiments of what today are organs of growth, metabolism and reproduction. We were transforming the elements of the sense organs from Saturn, some of which maintained their character, while others were transformed into glands and organs of growth[19].

The 'Sun' then passed into a sleep-condition again and was transformed into what we in occult science call the:

---

[19] We have completed two Days of Creation, which in the esoteric language are called: **Dies Saturni Dies Solis**. To them we must add: **Dies Lunae** (the Moon-Day). The existence of a directing Godhead of Saturn, Sun and Moon has always been known. The words Dies = Day and Deus = God have the same origin, so that Dies may be translated either Day or Godhead. One can just as well say for Dies Solis Sun-Day or Sun-God and mean by both translations the 'Christ Spirit'.

- **'Moon-evolution'**: This is the third incarnation of the 'Earth', which introduces us to a development that is of the utmost importance for the animal kingdom, the etheric body and the understanding of how diseases can translocate from humans to animals.

The development of the animals.
We will, in relation to the animals, try to start with the beginning, and then we relate our narrative to the cosmos of Rudolf Steiner.
The beginning of the creation of the higher animals started on the 'Old Moon', with the development of what has been called the "animal-man"-creatures. When present day earth developed, the less developed part of the animal-man population did not wait long enough for proper human forms to develop, and incarnated in animal forms. They were thus trapped in these bodies. The more developed souls waited until the bodily forms were mature enough to receive a being that could incarnate an "I-consciousness". These souls became men, the human kingdom. The human archetype waited for a much longer time in the spiritual world until it found a body mature enough to incarnate in. The less developed humans entered these immature forms which could not support an "I"-being. These beings then had to leave their spiritual "I" in the spiritual world, and this "I-consciousness then stayed in the spiritual world as the "I" of the group soul of that particular animal species.

Rudolf Steiner said in 1904 (and I repeat):
… simultaneously with its first incarnation in the beginning of the Lemurian age, the untarnished human spirit ….. sought its primal physical incarnation. The physical development of the earth with its animal-like creatures had not evolved so far at that time that it could incarnate the human spirit, the human "I". But a part of it, a certain group of animal-like beings had evolved so far

that the seed of the human spirit could descend into it to give form to the human body" (Steiner GA 93, 1904).

Edgar Cayce has a quite special story of the beginning, in which the first humans came down into the flesh, somewhat prematurely. According to Cayce the first men came down to earth prematurely, because they were tempted by the experiences of the flesh, especially the sexual experiences. They then became trapped in the material realm, although that was something they did not intend. They intended to just stay here for a short while. In the Bible they were then called the sons and daughters of man (Genesis 6, 1-6[20]).

Consequently, a rescue team was then sent down by a command of God the Creator, to lead the fallen men (those that had fallen into animal forms) back to God again, and so we have the present

---

[20] **The Bible** say the following:

Genesis 6 King James Version (KJV)

6 And it came to pass, when men began to multiply on the face of the earth, and daughters were born unto them,

[2] That the sons of God saw the daughters of men that they were fair; and they took them wives of all which they chose.

[3] And the Lord said, My spirit shall not always strive with man, for that he also is flesh: yet his days shall be an hundred and twenty years.

[4] There were giants in the earth in those days; and also after that, when the sons of God came in unto the daughters of men, and they bare children to them, the same became mighty men which were of old, men of renown.

[5] And God saw that the wickedness of man was great in the earth, and that every imagination of the thoughts of his heart was only evil continually.

[6] And it repented the Lord that he had made man on the earth, and it grieved him at his heart.

[7] And the Lord said, I will destroy man whom I have created from the face of the earth; both man, and beast, and the creeping thing, and the fowls of the air; for it repenteth me that I have made them.

[8] But Noah found grace in the eyes of the Lord.

[9] These are the generations of Noah: Noah was a just man and perfect in his generations, and Noah walked with God.

situation today where the animal kingdom must be rescued by the human kingdom.

A solution to liberate the souls entangled in matter was created by the spiritual world. First a physical form became available as a vehicle for the rescue-party-souls descending to Earth. Thus, a way was created for these souls to enter the Earth and experience it as part of their evolutionary/reincarnation cycle. Of the physical forms already existing on Earth, a species of anthropoid ape-man was the most appropriate to fulfil the required bodily form. Souls descended on these apes - hovering above and around them rather than inhabiting them, and influenced them to move towards a different goal from the simple one they had been pursuing. They left their tree habitations, built fires, made tools, lived in communities and began to communicate with one another. Eventually they lost their animal look, shed bodily hair, and took on refinements of manner and habit. The evolution of the human body occurred partly through the soul's influence on the endocrine glands until the ape-man was a three-dimensional objectification of the soul hovering above it. In this manner the soul fully descended into the physical body giving the Earth a new inhabitant: 'Homo sapiens'. Homo sapiens appeared in five different places on Earth at the same time, creating the five races we know today. This evolved human is what the Bible refers to as "Adam". When souls incarnated into physical form, it brought divine consciousness (i.e., the spirit) with it. Cayce referred to this divine consciousness as the "Christ Consciousness" or "Buddhahood" or the "super consciousness". Christ consciousness has little to do with the personality known as Jesus. It means a person has attained a complete human-divine unity. This human-divine unity has been attained by many people thus far - one such person was Jesus. The problem for the soul entangled in flesh was to overcome the attractions of the Earth to the extent the soul would be as free in the body as out of it. Only when the body was no longer a hindrance to the free expression of the soul could the cycle of Earth be finished. This is the condition of having a perfect unity of the human with the divine. In a smaller field, this was the evolutionary drama of free will and creation. In a still smaller field, each atom of the physical body is a world unto itself where a drama of free will and creation is occurring. The soul brings life into each atom, and each atom is a physical reflection of the soul's pattern. With the advent of consciousness, humans became aware of the sexual act meaning something more to them than to that of the animals. Sexual activity is the "door" which new souls enter the Earth, a door which is unnecessary in other heavenly planetary/realms. Sexual activity is thus the only means which trapped souls have of being liberated from their predicament - through the cycle of birth, death and rebirth.

I will here refer to a special reading by Edgar Cayce (numbered after his special system):

A 1936 reading (1183-1) mentioned giants in Lemuria. According to Cayce, Lemuria, or Mu, was a land based in the South Pacific that was all but destroyed by 50,000 B.C. Cayce related that there were many changes happening to the physical surface of the Earth at that time (upheavals and natural disasters) and that the "sons and daughters of men" were interacting with "the sons of the daughters of God." According to the reading, many thought forms were projecting themselves into physical form on Earth and that "monsters" were present. Many of these were large, dangerous animals that roamed in large herds that caused destruction. Most Cayce scholars believe he was referring to mastodons, mammoths, and mega-fauna such as saber tooth tigers and giant sloth. But various readings refer to "things"—animal monstrosities. In some readings Cayce related that various "things" were created by what appears to be some form of genetic manipulation. The 1936 reading tells us that this was the time period related to in the biblical quote: "in those days there were giants in the earth." The use of the terms "sons and daughters of men" and "sons and daughters of God" are apparently unique to Cayce, but he described the meaning of these terms in various places. Human life, according to Cayce, resulted from thought forms (souls) that moved into the universe and projected themselves into physical form. But by so doing, the energy-based soul becomes trapped in physical matter. Cayce's term "sons and daughters of men" refers to "souls who had become so physical, so terrestrial as to have lost their awareness" (Edgar Cayce's Atlantis; 2006; Little, Van Auken, & Little). In losing this awareness of their true spiritual nature, the souls were destined to reincarnate into physical form until they regained their awareness of their nature and origin. The "sons and daughters of men" had evolved over many lifetimes and became physically smaller in size. But during this early time period, somewhere around 210,000 B.C., more thought forms projected into physical form and they initially retained some of their awareness about their true nature. These were called the "sons and daughters of God" because they still had a connection to their source and remained somewhat god-like. Trapped within their encasement in physical form, the "daughters of men" began to interbreed with the newly arriving "sons of God" "creating creatures that were half god-like in their size and power and half human." These were referred to in the Bible as the Nephilim. Inca legends tell of a time when bands of these gigantic, half-breed offspring came to the shores of their land causing havoc until natural forces arose and ridded the land of them. Many Native American legends also tell of the arrival of giants that were cannibals who eventually became rulers.

We see from this that both animals and man originate from the same souls.
The only difference being that some souls were too eager to descend into the physical and material world.
They were trapped in animal forms and became the higher animals.
They are our brothers and sisters, and it is our duty to help them become human one day.

We must and should treat them with love and respect.

The animals are our brothers and sisters, our lost siblings, and they are connected to our future whether we like it or not.

Every species has their own "I" in the spiritual world that is functioning in their group-soul.

Each human being has their own "I" while every animal species has their common "I" in the higher spiritual world.

Each human being has their own astral body, while the animal species have their specific "group-soul" in the upper part of the earth´s atmosphere.

Every individual animal has an astral body that is a concentrated aspect of the group-soul, in which each individual animal soul participates. The repertoire of emotions which are available to each animal comes from the group-soul, and what each individual animal experiences returns to the group soul.

More about the group-soul in animals:

In 1924 Rudolf Steiner wrote:

> ……….. what is it that we call instinct in the animals? We know that the animals have a Group-soul. The animal, such as it is, is not a self-contained being. The Group-soul is standing there behind it. Now to what world does the Group-soul belong? We must first answer this question: Where do we find the Group-souls of the animals? They are certainly not to be found here in the physical world of sense. Here we have only the single individual animals. We do not find the Group-souls of the animals until, by Initiation or in the ordinary course of human evolution between death and a new birth, we come into that altogether different world which man passes through

between his successive earthly lives. There indeed we find, among the beings with whom we are then together, including above all those of whom I have been speaking to you, those with whom we elaborate our karma, — there we find the Group-souls of the animals. And the animals that are here on the earth, when they act instinctively, they act out of the full consciousness of the Group-souls. You may conceive it thus, my dear friends. (Dr. Steiner here made a drawing on the blackboard). Here we have the realm in which we live between death and a new birth; and out of it there work the forces which proceed from the Group-souls of the animals. And here upon this earth we have the single animals which act and move about, guided as it were by threads which pass to the Group-souls — the beings whom we ourselves discover in the realm between death and a new birth. Such in truth is instinct. It is obvious that a materialistic world-conception cannot explain instinct, for instinct is: — to act out of that sphere of being which you will find described as Spirit-land in my **Theosophy** *for example, and in my* **Occult Science**. *For man however it is different. Man too has instinct, but when he acts through his instinct, he is not acting out of yonder Spirit-realm, but out of his own former lives on earth. He is acting across time, out of his former earthly lives, out of a whole number of former lives on earth. As the spiritual realm works upon the animals, causing them to act instinctively, so do the former incarnations of man work on his later incarnations in such a way that he instinctively lives out his karma. But this is a spiritual instinct — an instinct that works within the Ego. It is just by understanding this, that we shall come to understand the absolute consistency of this instinctive working with human freedom. For the freedom of man proceeds from the very realm out of which the animals act instinctively, namely the realm of the spirit. Today we will concern ourselves especially with* *the way in which this instinct is gradually prepared when man passes through the gate of death. Here in earthly life, as we have seen, the inner experience of karma is instinctive. It takes its course beneath the surface of consciousness; but the moment we pass through the gate of death we become objectively conscious, during the first few days, of all the experiences which we first underwent on earth. We have them before us in ever expanding pictures; and what we thus behold as a great tableau of our life contains, in addition, all that took place instinctively in the working of our karma.[21]*

The beginning of an individual "I" in animals.
If the group-soul has opened up to the human being, either individually (seldom) or as a group (usual), the species is called 'tame', or domesticated. Being 'domesticated' implies that the group-soul has opened itself to the human "I". This opening up affects all the individuals in a species, with the exception of those members of the species that have been met with too much violence from human interaction, thus closing their 'individual openings'.

This opening of the animal group-soul for the human being, for the human "I", also means that parts of, or rather a 'mirror-image' of the human "I" is projected into the specific animal. It is as if the group soul has opened to a general influx of human soul- and "I"-properties.

This I have witnessed myself.

I had during the years 2005 till 2010 a horse named "Balder". He was a gelding of North-Swedish heritage, a firm and typically cold-blooded horse. I was closely attached to him and loved him dearly. It felt as though we could read each other's thoughts. After a long

---

[21] Lecture by Rudolf Steiner, 4th of July 1924, (GA 237).

and chronic disease, I had to shoot him at the farm where we both had lived for some years. At the spot where he was shot I could both see him (his spiritual entity) and follow his 'path' for several days. The first two days he was sort of angry with me for having taken his life. Then he went into his own 'purgatorio', where he fought with etheric wolves for two days. This was his deep-rooted fear, actually the fear of all horses, and after death they experience this vividly. Then a most interesting thing happened. A mare of Hannoveranian breed happened to pass by. This mare also lived at our farm, and she was inseminated just a few days earlier with sperm from one of Germanys best Hannoveranian stallions. When the mare passed by the whole etheric/astral soul of Balder dissolved in a sort of mist, and this mist streamed or flowed into the stomach of the mare.

Nine months went by, and the foal was born under the Hannoveranian mare. My x-wife, who was very skilled in horse-breeding and a connoisseur of horse races, was shocked. The foal was like a 50/50 % mix of cold-blood and Hannoveranian.

My conclusion of this happening was that due to love between Balder and me, which must have involved some kind of individual soul pattern, he was able to withstand the call of the group-soul and incarnate in a somewhat different race just to continue to be close to me.

We see here how the close relationship and love between humans and animals will and can lay the foundation of the development of both an individual soul (separated from the group) and an individual "I"-consciousness that can even re-incarnate.

Many dog owners and their families have also observed how dogs more and more take over their master's individuality. This phenomenon has to be discussed more in length, as it differs somewhat from the teachings of Rudolf Steiner (as far as I know).

Rudolf Steiner describes a "normal" change in the animals that have a certain "I"-consciousness or individualized group-soul after death as follows.

In 1908 Rudolf Steiner wrote:

> Just as this describes what we begin to feel with regard to these unsuspected beings, so it is where the souls of the plants are concerned. The plant egos dwell in a higher world than the animal egos. The separate group egos of the plants live on what we call the devachanic plane. We can even state the place where they actually are — in the very center of the earth, whereas the animal group souls circle round the earth like trade winds. All these plant egos at the center point of the earth are mutually interpenetrating beings, for in the spiritual world a law of penetrability prevails and all beings pass through one another. We see the animal group souls moving over the earth like trade winds, and how in their wisdom they carry out what appears to be done by the animals. Studying the plant, we see that its head — the root — is directed towards the center of the earth where its group ego is to be found. The earth itself is the outward expression of soul and spirit beings. From the spiritual point of view the plants seem like the nails of our fingers. The plants belong to the earth, and when we look at them singly we do not see a complete entity, for the single plant is just one among the whole number of beings constituting a group ego. In this way we can enter into what the plants themselves feel. The part of the plant that springs up out of the earth, what from within the earth strives up to the surface, is of a different nature from what is growing under the earth. There is a difference between the cutting off of blossoms, stalk, leaves, and the tearing up of a root. The former gives the plant soul a feeling of well-being, of pleasure, just as it gives pleasure to a cow, for example, when the calf sucks milk from her udder. There is actual similarity between the milk of animals,

and that part of a plant which pushes its way out of the earth. When in late summer we go through fields where corn is being cut, where the blade is passing through the corn stems, then the whole fields breathe out a feeling of bliss. It is an intensely significant moment when we not only watch the reaping with our physical eyes, but perceive the feeling of contentment sweeping over the earth as the corn falls to the ground. But when the roots of the plants are pulled up, then that is painful for the plant souls. In the higher worlds the same laws do not hold good which are valid in the physical world. When we rise to the spiritual worlds our conceptions become different; even here on the physical plane there is sometimes opposition between the principle of beauty and that of pain or pleasure. It is possible that, impelled by a feeling for beauty, someone might pull out their white hairs, that indeed would be painful. And it is like that in the case of the plants. When the roots are pulled up this may make for neatness — yet the plants suffer. Even stone is without life only on the physical plane. All minerals have their group egos in the higher worlds, on the higher devachanic plane, and these, too, feel pain and pleasure. Only spiritual science can teach us about these matters; speculation is of no avail. Looking at a quarry, and watching the splitting off of each block of stone, one might imagine this to cause pain for the stone ego. But it is not so. With the actual splitting of stone, there gushes out in all directions a feeling of pleasure. Out of the quarry from which the blocks are being cut, there streams deep satisfaction on every side. And if we put salt into a glass of water so that it dissolves, then, too, a feeling of pleasure flows through the water. We see this pleasure stream through the water if, with eyes of the spirit, we watch the salt dissolve; but when the salt is becoming crystallized again the pleasure turns to pain. And it would be painful for the stone ego were we able to remold the severed blocks into their original bed (Rudolf Steiner, THE

GROUP SOULS OF ANIMALS, PLANTS AND MINERALS, Frankfurt-am-Main, 2nd February, 1908).

We will now try to imagine the animal group-soul, and also the animal group-"I", and compare it to the human soul and "I", and how these interact with each other when there arises love between an animal and a human being.

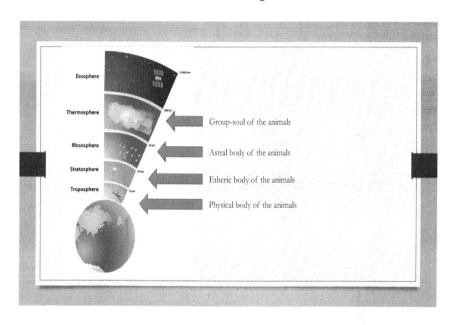

There has been a multitude of observations in how different animal species can communicate, talk, remember and reason.
This is especially seen in the great apes, with birds like ravens and crows, in elephants, whales and in dolphins.

Many of these animals also have the ability to recognize themselves in a mirror.

All humans that have owned and loved a dog, a cat or a horse know that they too have their own individuality.

Many different observations have shown that animals can have a certain "I"-function. There are equally as many that point to the fact that they don't.

All of these controversies and differing opinions and observations can be solved by accepting the possibility of translocation.

Human diseases can enter animals through the multiplying 'demon' of the disease. This also applies to translocated parts or reflections of these parts as well as smaller copies of the human "I"-function through the human-animal connection, especially furthered by love between a human and an animal.

When the animal group-soul becomes 'tamed', it opens up to the human soul, and also to the human "I". The animal species as a whole open up to the dominion of humans, and accept the 'taming process'. This bring them the possibility of receiving all the human diseases as well as bringing into being the beginning of the individual soul and the individual "I"-consciousness.

We must again remember what Edgar Cayce described, that several of the higher animals actually inhabit human souls, or at least human souls that *'should'* have been human, but due to their eagerness and impatience became trapped in animal bodies. In these 'human-animal' bodies it is possible for shamans to incarnate as the bodies of these animals are 'familiar' with a human-like soul. If we examine the stories of indigenous people world over, they are capable of incarnating in large birds, horses and wolves. I have personally never heard about shamanic incarnations in dolphins or whales. The only time I myself have experienced incarnation in an animal was in a bird, and it was actually quite pleasant, apart from all the troubles I had with managing the big beak. It was always in the way[22].

---

[22] This is described in my book «*The forgotten mysteries of Atlantis*», published on Amazon.com.

The animals are thus highly sentient beings, having a common group-soul, as well as a "group"-"I" and a slightly emerging individual sentient soul along with an emerging "I"-consciousness, linked with and dependent on the human soul- and "I"-consciousness.

Scientists of today are accepting more and more that animals have highly developed feelings, possibly even higher than humans, and that they may indeed have entirely different feelings than us.
This is an extremely important part of animal behavior and disease. The owner and the veterinarian often overlook or at least underestimate the sentient ability of animals.

There is also evidence that some animals, especially dogs and cats, dream. Usually we admit that animals have feelings like fear and aggression, but many researchers believe that animals have the whole range of feelings, just as humans, maybe even more.

According to Rudolf Steiner animals experience *more* pain than humans:

In 1910 Rudolf Steiner wrote:

> So we understand "pain" in the astral body by conceiving it as the expression of weakness of the etheric body in relation to the physical body. An etheric body that is in harmony with its physical body works back upon the astral body in such a way that the feeling of well-being is an inner experience of health. On the other hand, an etheric body that is at odds with its physical body works back upon the astral body in such a way that pain and discomfort are bound to arise in it. Now we shall be able to realize that because in the higher animals — it will be better to speak of the lower animals in the next lecture — the life of soul is so intimately bound up with the bodily nature, this soul experience will be much more deeply felt

— as will also be the case in a disordered body — than it can be in a disordered human body. Because the soul life of man is emancipated from the inner, bodily experience, pain that is merely due to bodily circumstances is far less torturing, it gnaws much less deeply into the soul than in the higher animals. We can also observe that bodily pain in children is a much keener psychic pain than in later life, because in the measure in which the adult human being becomes independent of his bodily organization, he finds in the qualities which arise immediately out of his soul, the means to struggle against bodily pain; whereas the higher animal, being so closely bound up with its bodily nature, feels pain with infinitely greater intensity than man. Those who maintain that human pain can be more intense than pain felt by the animals, are talking without foundation. Pain in the animal is far, far more deep-seated than purely bodily pain in man can ever be (Rudolf Steiner 10th of November 1910, GA 60).

These include feelings like sorrow, joy, depression, elation, grief, compassion, melancholy, longing etc. They may even have feelings that we do not understand or cannot imagine, since we may not have the full range of animal feelings.

I have often observed how the emotions of the keeper or stable-girl have influenced the animals through the whole day. Many farmers report that the frequency of mastitis increases when they have weekend-help in the barn. It can be very stressful for cows to be milked by an unknown and insensitive person. The stress reaction can precipitate immunosuppression, which can allow mastitis to arise.

I have noted that a change of staff or riders often is associated with decreased performance in thoroughbred horses. This is especially marked when former staff or riders had a close and good relationship with the horses and maybe even worked overtime to make life easier for them. I have noted a long-lasting decrease in racing ability, and more infections and injuries, when regular known staff is replaced with someone that is much tougher or heavy handed.

I will, to demonstrate the advanced sensitivity of the animals, cite the following:

Two examples from my practice:

- A Norwegian horse was to be sold in Germany. At home it showed no lameness and was a very stable and friendly horse. But as soon as it arrived in Germany it became lame, got bruises, wounds and other serious problems. It was not sold. By chance I was in the area and had the opportunity to treat the horse. In investigating the animal with the help of Pulse Diagnosis, I found the energy in the HT meridian to be almost zero. The horse showed severe signs of sorrow, knowing it was to be sold. I treated the HT meridian, and the horse changed radically, and all the problems vanished like dew to the sun. As the owner realized this connection, she immediately took the horse home again to Norway.
- Another horse was to be sold, and it had been free of problems for a long time, but on examination in Oslo it showed severe lameness in several legs. It was sent to my clinic where I found a severe Qi deficiency in the HT meridian (via Pulse Diagnosis), which led to a decreased blood circulation in the front legs. The horse had mourned being sold, and developed what we in humans call a bruised and broken heart. The horse was treated, and all the problems disappeared quickly.

I have also noticed that noise from fans, bad smell from manure, humidity due to bad ventilation, irregular feeding and careless husbandry, highly influence meat or milk quality,

In the more relaxed and easygoing days, the old farmers in the West of Ireland had a saying "Look after your animals and they will look after you". Compassion towards animals involves treating animals as individuals, treating them with respect, dignity, patience, gentleness and kindness. It also involves close physical contact (massaging, scratching and rubbing the animals), talking and singing to them, and *playing with them*. Today, these aspects of animal care are not taken as seriously as they should be. The reasons for this are multiple. One reason is that modern labor is scarce and expensive. One worker must handle many more animals today than was the case in the past. Therefore, animal handlers do not have the time to get to know the individual natures, likes and dislikes of their animals. Even if they do know, they cannot, or will not, take the time to cater for individual needs or preferences in their animals.

Another important factor is that quantity rather than quality is the measure of animal productivity today. This is not so obvious in pork meat (even though many studies show the relationship between stress and meat quality) as in the objectively recorded race times in horses. Race times certainly become longer in stressed animals.

Death of animals as compared to humans and plants.
Here I will start by citing what Rudolf Steiner has said about this matter.

In 1912 Rudolf Steiner said:

> *"How are we to conceive that the plants begin and end their existence? How are we to picture, so to speak, the birth and death of a plant? We shall see at once that these words applied to the plant kingdom have, fundamentally, no more real significance than if we were to say, when a man's hair falls out that the hair is dead. Once a man rises to the thought that with regard to the earth he is dealing with an ensouled organism, he acquires a completely new outlook on the beginning and end of life in the plant world. To anyone not merely following the single plant individual purely externally, from seed to seed again, but rather bearing in mind the sum total of plant life on the earth, it will be obvious that here something different is at work from what may be called the beginning and end of life in*

*the animal, or the human, kingdom .... for the life of the earth is in the season from autumn to spring. Hence, we cannot speak of a real death or a real birth in plants at all, only of a sleeping and waking of the whole earth organism. As in human beings sleeping and waking is repeated rhythmically in the course of twenty-four hours, and as we do not speak in this connection of the death and birth of our thought world either, if we wish to speak correctly, should we speak of the life and death of plants. We should keep the whole earth organism in view, regarding the plant process belonging to the whole earth organism as a waking up and falling asleep of the earth ......
Now let us try to investigate what we can call death in the animal kingdom, not indeed by making judgments through analogy but rather, by expressing once more, through a process in the human being, what Spiritual Science has to give .... all that is feeling and passion in the whole earth organism is lived out in the animal kingdom just as our passions and impulses are lived out in our whole organization. As we look at the animal world we see in each separate form the result of the disposition of the soul of our earth. And if we consider the attraction which the earth exercises over the life of the animal world, allowing itself to be most closely linked with the external physical body, we see that this is no other than the victory of the spiritual — of what, with regard to animals we call the group soul. It is the super-sensible element which finds its representative only in externals, and conquers the external, as in man the spiritual feelings conquer what is merely instinctive. That the external processes of the earth organization always acquiesce in the power of death over the individual animal is in no way different from the victory always achieved in us by the spiritual over what is merely connected with the organic. Seeing the spiritual element in the animal from this point of view, we cannot apply the expressions birth and death to the beginning and end of an*

animal's existence in the same way as we apply them to man. It is certainly in animals a process of the whole earth, already more individualized than in the plant world. Nevertheless, if we bear in mind the different group souls assigned to the various animal species, we must see how, in each death which overtakes the individual animal, the external, bodily part perishes, but the group soul, which is the spiritual element in the animal, is always triumphant over the external form; just as in man the spiritual triumphs over the merely instinctive, represented not in the separate form but certainly in the organization. Thus we see, as it were, a vast living being composed of the individual group souls of the animals, and we see the birth and death of the living animal appear in such a way that what forms the foundation of the spiritual in the individual animal has always to fight for its victory over the individuality. Hence, we have death in animals presented as that which, as the group soul, moves above the wasting and decay of the individual animal form. We could only speak of a real death in connection with an animal if we failed to bear in mind what remains after the death of an animal; namely, the spiritual, as in man the spiritual, rising above itself, triumphs over the disposition of soul as well as over what is doomed to wither away. — If Darwinism ever advances beyond its present stage, it will see how, throughout the animal kingdom, from the earliest ages, a thread of evolution runs through the apparent births and deaths into the distant future; so that the whole evolution of the animal kingdom will lead at last to a victory of what the lower, the individual animal form being overcome — will issue from the entire spiritual world, leaving behind the lower part living in the individual animals, and will one day triumph over the instinctive element apparent in the whole of animal nature.

And when in man we come to what we call the human will nature — if we then do not speak only of the ideas he has had, which can be recalled again and again, and do not fix our attention only on the soul disposition which sinks in the way described into the deeper organization — if we, rather, look to the impulses of the will, we shall see that they represent above all the most enigmatic part of human nature. How the impulses of a man's will are determined depends upon the experiences life has brought him. If we look back from any point in our life, we find a continuous path, a movement, in which each soul event is linked with one before it. We find, however, that what we have experienced flows mainly into our will in such a way that if we look at ourselves thus, we may say that we have actually become richer in ideas, and riper with respect to the impulses of our will. Indeed, we develop a very special ripeness with respect to our will. This is experienced by everyone looking back upon his life .... an animal's death is quite different from that of a man. In the case of man death has to do with the bringing down of his individual ego on to the physical plane and the identification of it with his physical body. A man speaks of his physical body as "I" — feels himself to be "I". When at death he loses his physical body it is a perceptible process, and he feels he is losing something of value. For those accustomed to look upon the physical body as valueless, the loss is less severe. The single animal has no such sense of "I am". That is experienced by the group soul. The more a being is individualized, and the deeper its descent on the physical plane, the more difficult its regeneration becomes. The group soul feels the death of an animal as we should the loss of a finger — as something to be compensated for or replaced. After long periods the animals on earth change. Species evolve. Darwinism has elaborated this hypothetically, but the following is really the case. When

*an animal species changes there is also a change of group
soul; and when the species becomes extinct this, for the
group soul, is similar to death. For example, the seer today
can discern a kind of death rattle in the group soul of the
ibex. But the group soul evolves and becomes, on the
extinction of one animal species, the group soul of another
— which is like a rebirth[23].*

The functional mechanisms of translocation.

Now, after understanding the development and construction of
both the universe, of man and of animals, how they live, how they
die and how they connect to the human beings, it will be easier to
understand the mechanism of translocation.

One interesting aspect of translocation is that the pathological
entity, demon, specter or phantom, almost always goes from the
stronger entity to the weaker, and when it goes to this weaker
entity, there must be a place for it to lodge, a void in which it can
find its space, its house.

In an animal that is tamed, one that has opened its 'group-soul' to
mankind, either to humans in general or to a specific human, then
the "I" of the human being is always stronger that the 'part-group-
soul' that the animal possesses. When the animal undergoes some
kind of stress or receives insufficient food, the animal then
provides a void in which a part of the demon based in the human
being can enter. The 'human demon' splits off a clone, and this
clone then enters the animal and becomes an 'animal demon'.

In this way the animal also brings the 'demon-clone' in contact with
the whole group-soul, thus one single human may 'infect' a whole
group of animals.

---

[23] Lecture held by Rudolf Steiner, "Der Tod bei Mench, Tier und Pflantze",
Berlin, 29th of February, 1912 (GA 61).

An example:
Once I was called by a sheep farmer living in the upper part of Gudbrandsdalen in Norway. All of his 80 sheep had got the same problem, a definite problem with the estrus cycle, the reproductive cycle. This occurred immediately after he had hired a new shepherdess who had come up from Oslo. He called me to ask for advice concerning his sick sheep. I immediately felt that this disease was not due to some estrogen containing herb, it was due to translocation from a human. I asked to talk with the shepherdess, and became convinced that her menstrual and hormonal problems were the cause. I asked her to return to Oslo, and as soon as she did this the problem disappeared.
Nothing else was changed.

An example:
I had been asked to treat a young woman with cystitis, bladder infection. She was 30 years of age, and had suffered from a chronic cystitis for 25 years. She came together with her mother, a very special woman of 50 years. Through pulse-diagnosis I found the deficiency (treated after the 5-element thinking, a thinking which I now know furthers translocation instead of transformation), and treated her bladder. All the time while I was with the 25 years old woman, the mother was speaking about herself, how she also had been suffering from chronic cystitis for decades. It was me, me, me and me. A few days later I was called by the mother saying that her daughter was not better, but that she was totally cured. I was astonished, asked her daughter to come back without her, and after treating the daughter alone she also was cured.

An example:
A man from Oslo brought me two small dogs that had a chronic pruritus (scratching) that nobody had been able to cure, not "even" at the veterinary high school. I pulsed both dogs, and found that each had a heart deficiency. I then turned to the owner and pulsed him, and found that he also had a heart deficiency. On asking him how long the two dogs had been suffering from the eczema, he

answered two years. I asked who had left him and caused him heartbreak about 2 years ago, upon which he almost burst into tears telling me that the love of his life had left him just a month before both dogs begun suffering from eczema. I then treated the owners heart meridian, also asking him to deal with his sorrow and talk with the lost love, and after 2 weeks both dogs were 90% better.

An example:
A German dressage horse had a severe problem in turning right for 2 years. Many veterinarians, osteopaths, acupuncturists and chiropractics had tried to treat the horse, but without success. The horse did not get better. I asked the rider if I could examine her (the rider herself), and found a stuck vertebrae (C4) in her neck. I manipulated the vertebrae, and right after asked her to test the horse again. She protested as I hadn't even touched the horse, but after my insisting questioning she accepted to try the horse. She put the saddle on and rode out into the riding house. 10 minutes later she came back. The horse was then 100% cured.

An example:
There is an epidemy of mammary cancer today in dogs. Likewise, there is a steadily growing number of women that get breast cancer. This is for me, and should be for many, a very obvious example of translocation.

Of course, such examples referred to here can be explained in other ways, all of them. But if you really *see* the demonic translocation, other explanations seem silly and just uninteresting.

The spatial mechanism of human-animal translocation.
One may consider the 'tame' animals as having allowed the human spirit and soul, yes actually the whole human spiritual makeup, to enter or communicate with both their individual soul and their group-soul. When a whole species (as the cows) have opened their

group-soul to the influence of humans, all cows will submit to the human will, thoughts and feelings. The individual animal reflects this opening, and lets the specific owner or care-giver influence it. This is an opening in the group-soul, in the collective group-soul, and as such all animals of the species will accept the dominion of the humans. This mechanism was demonstrated by the sheep-herd in Gudbrandsdalen, in Norway, referred to earlier. The influence or passage-way goes from the human "I"-consciousness to the animal "group-soul". Such a passage always goes from above to below, from the "I" to the astral body, from the astral to the etheric and from the etheric to the physical.

In humans the diseases or moods in a grown-up's astral body will influence the children's etheric body, very important to know for parents and teachers.

In animals their group-soul will always be influenced by the "I" of the humans. That is why humans seldom get influenced by animals. It is of course possible that the pathology of the group-soul or the astral body of the animal can slip into the etheric body of a human being, causing the human being to become immediately sick (zoonoses). I saw this once at a seminar in Worpswede (Germany), I treated a horse from the Middle-Point with Christ-Consciousness. After the treatment "something" came out of the horse, and this "something" swirled around inside the circle of watching students. They should not have been standing in a circle, as that captured the "something" (as described in the beginning of Goethe's 'Faust', when Mephistopheles is ensnared in a circle drawn on the floor by Faustus). Then it (the 'something') disappeared into thin air. One of the students happened to attract a part of the "something" that was released. Returning home after the seminar she immediately became sick. Thanks to her therapist who was able to quickly diagnose this "partial pathological structure" and release it, she recovered without serious damage (how that was done I do not know, it was probably translocated further).

The "something" was stuck in her heart, where it tried to make its new home.

If we consider the animal soul and group-soul as related to the earth and its atmosphere, we find that the group-soul is situated in the 'thermosphere' of the earth, some 80 – 1000 kilometer above the surface of the earth, where the physical bodies of the animals are dwelling. It is in this height that the human pathological entities or demons enter the animal. This might seem a little strange, but the following story will perhaps make this more probable.

While working in Northern-Norway I had some communication with the Sami people.

The Sami people have a huge knowledge about the 'Aurora Borealis', also called the 'Northern Light'. They believe, actually they "know", that the Aurora can make you crazy, that it can enter your body, and all children are warned to be cautious. I was also told that if you had a certain feeling for animals, you could 'direct' the Aurora at your wish. You just had to attract its awareness, its astral awareness, and then it would follow your wishes or directions. One night, in the darkness of the north, I was the last passenger on a boat home from a visit to a sick cow. I was in the company of a Sami man, who showed me the secret techniques of directing the Aurora.

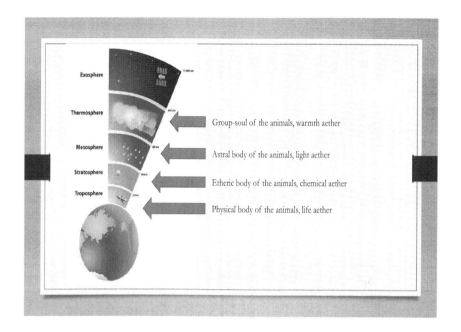

It was unbelievable! I made the Aurora go where I wanted it to go, to behave as I wanted. It was totally at my command. I realized that the Aurora was 800000 meters up in the air, and found the experience quite astonishing. This indicates that the activity in the Thermosphere is in direct contact with our "I"-consciousness, and that this consciousness can have full connection with the animalistic forces of that area, the animal group-souls.

It is important to know that the connection between humans and animals encompass the whole earth and its atmosphere up to 100 kilometers, including also the possibility to influence the weather.

It is also very interesting to be aware of the temperature in the area of the atmosphere where the intervention between the human "I" and the animal group-soul takes place. We normally believe or think that the higher we get the colder it gets. This is not so. From the surface of the earth it gets colder and colder the higher we go, but at some point, it starts to get warmer.

At about 20 km above the earth, at the ending of the troposphere it is very cold, around -60 degree Celsius. When we go further we reach the ozone layer in the stratosphere, about 50000 meters up, and there the temperature is around 0 degrees. Then when reaching a height of about 80000 meters, at the beginning of the thermosphere it sinks to -40 again. Reaching the middle of the thermosphere the temperature may reach +1500 degrees Celsius, very warm indeed. In this temperature the northern lights, the aurora borealis play out it might, and here the full interconnection between humans and animals take place. That is why the human "I" can fully and totally interfere and dominate the fluctuations of the Aurora.

A thought: Could our present cruel treatment of the animals have anything to do with the climate crisis???????

All disease-creating demons (ahrimanic), specters (luciferic) or phantoms (azuric) can either be translocated or transformed.

The strongest transforming force is love.

This chapter uncovers the horrific mind shattering realization experienced by animal owners, human and veterinary therapists, when they come to understand the full impact that pathological entities called demons, specters or phantoms, can or will be translocated to other beings through the treatment of a 5-element based energetic method, which includes 'school-medicine' and several other healing methods based on 'natural medical methods'.

Translocation vs Transformation.
I have observed when treating patients, there are two fundamental methods of treatment.

- Treating the excess, the symptoms.
- Treating the deficiency, the root cause of the disease.

The first method, used widely in allopathic medicine, treats the symptoms directly. For example, one reduces a fever by giving anti-inflammatories, cooling herbs, or heat dispelling acupuncture points. I have termed this method of translocation as *treating the excess.*

Or, the healer can attempt to treat at a deeper level, more commonly used in alternative medicine, by stimulating the vital force. That is, to treat the underlying fundamental weakness that created the symptoms in the first place. I have termed this as *treating the deficiency.* Earlier in my career as a healer, I was under the assumption that the later was the superior and more curative method. I now realize that both techniques are suboptimal, as with both modalities, the pathological entity is simply transposed to another host. However, the treatment of the excess translocates 90% of the diseases, whereas the treatment of the deficiency translocates only 40 % of the diseases[24]. It has only been in the last few years of my practice that I have come to this realization which showed itself through my treatment of cancer, described in detail later in this chapter. When my cancer treatments stopped working after 30 years of positive results (80% total healing and remission of the cancer), I had to question the deeper foundations of this treatment. I then knew that I had to find a method that could truly annihilate the disease, truly transform the disease, transform it to something good, something beneficial.

Introduction to my cancer therapy.

Three decades ago, when I began adopting the modalities of homeopathy and acupuncture, I enjoyed a substantial degree of success in helping my patients. I continued to increase the efficacy of these treatments by adding the innovative use of both acupuncture Ting-points to treat equine pathology (1982) and the control cycle of five element acupuncture in the treatment of cancer in both humans and animals (1984).

However, later I came to the discovery that my treatments actually enforced a translocation of the disease to other persons and animals.[25] From my experience almost all diseases in animals are translocated from their owners in a "natural" way, but the traditional alternative treatment enforces this system. I gradually realized through both careful observation of pathological symptoms in whole families and also direct spiritual seeing that

---

[24] If a disease is translocated, this happens usually.

[25] This discovery was primarily made by seeing with my clairvoyant abilities that from childhood I have worked with and trained. I have written more about how to train clairvoyance in my books "Pappel" (Amazon), "Demons and Healing" (Temple Lodge), "Spiritual Medicine" (Amazon) and "Experiences from the Threshold" (Amazon).

the pathological entities that were causing the illness were not transformed, and that my earlier 'success' was not actually resulting in a true cure. In fact, I was merely exteriorizing these entities allowing their transmission to another host. Furthermore, I concluded that these adversaries were quite resistant to what I call transformation[26].

The process of transformation can be likened to disarming these noxious stimuli, rendering them free of malicious intent and rehabilitating them with qualities that will actually help rather than hinder mankind.

Observing my cancer treatments in 2014, I became acutely aware that the pathological entities just translocated to other hosts, which seemingly made my treatment easy and 'successful'.

Realizing that pathological entities were not so bothered about changing hosts I knew that I had to stop treating in this way and change my usual protocols, as I felt more and more un-ethical by translocating the diseases.

---

[26] As my studies of Anthroposophic Medicine evolved, I concluded that all chronic diseases in man are perpetuated by the inhabitancy of "Yin-pathological entities" (Ahrimanic) and "Yang-pathological entities" (Luciferic). These structures reside in separate regions of the body; the "Yang-pathological entities" in the cranial midsection, while the "Yin-pathological entities" in the caudal area of the body. I also discovered that the level of health of the patient was directly correlated to the distance between these two structures. In a relatively healthy state, the distance in a person approximates 20 cm, while in an average horse they are separated by as much as 80 cm. The closer the two entities migrate toward each other, the greater the pathology. Most importantly, I have "seen" that, in cancer, there is a minimal distance between the two, as if they have joined forces. Deductively, I concluded that the effect of these demons is exaggerated by their proximity to one another. As I started to "see" these structures more often with my spiritual eyes, I began to understand the importance of translocation in treatment. I realized that most diseases were being treated by addressing one of the two "pathological entities": either by weakening or opposing the "Yin-pathological entity" (treatment of the deficiency) or by weakening or opposing the "Yang-pathological entities" (treatment of the excess). I also discovered that both of these methods are more or less symptomatic, often just translocating the pathology to other places in the body or to other humans or animals.

Then came the crucial and important moment (March 2014) when I made the decision to *intend* and *want* to stop this translocation. At the same moment the effect of the cancer-treatment *more or less disappeared.*

The curative effect of my cancer treatment stopped. Not only for me, but also for most of my students. This happened at the same time, without anybody knowing about each other.

Since 2014 I have been working to restore the effect of my treatment without translocating the disease. Finally, in 2017, I began making headway towards a solution to this dilemma.

It is of crucial importance for this book to discuss, describe and understand the treatment protocols that one can use to enable transformation and the resultant true annihilation of the disease. As written earlier in this book, 95% of all internal diseases in animals originate from the owner. This phenomenon has also been described in many ancient texts such as the Bible. Therefore, once it becomes clear that the owner is translocating his disease to the animal it is necessary to treat both of them in order to truly transform the pathology in its entirety.

For example, I treated a woman with anxiety disorder and found that a few days later her dog stopped urinating in the house. This happened without directly treating the animal and therefore represented a truly transformative treatment for both of them. I have relayed this information in my courses and the feedback from my students and colleagues have substantiated this claim. Additionally, translocation can occur among the members of a household. For example, I have seen chronic cystitis in a female patient, only to observe the same pulse pathology and translocated prostatitis in her husband a few months later. However, by treating the wife and husband through transformational techniques both were cured. Without using the methods that facilitate transformation (a *cure*) we resort to accomplishing only one of three scenarios.

- First, we merely *palliate* the case as we watch its repeated return months or years later.
- Or, secondly, we *suppress* the disease by substituting a less sinister pathology with a much worse disease.
- Thirdly we can translocate the disease to another entity.

An example of the second possibility is the use of steroids to suppress an atopic dermatitis only to replace it with Cushing's disease later.

If one reviews the literature of various alternative medical systems, there are revelations that show that this translocation phenomena was already being observed in earlier times, especially by some of the great physicians of homeopathy, such as Dr. Constantine Hering, the author of Hering's Laws of Cure. The gold standard of the evidence of a cure was eloquently categorized by this physician as a centrifugal exteriorization of the symptoms from serious spiritual and organic disease to superficial areas such as the skin. The eventual positive outcome being a person with total freedom of body, mind, and spirit in order to enlist his higher calling. What was not overtly addressed in this law was the transmission of such demons to other beings on the planet. Therefore, in a global perspective, this does not represent a cure.

For the last 30 years, as both an anthroposophist, a veterinarian and an acupuncturist, I have tried to find methods of treatment that do not merely translocate, palliate or suppress the pathology, but rather result in a transformation in order to evoke a truly curative response. During my search, I gradually discovered that each "acupuncture technique" that I modified resulted in different effects on my patient as shown below:

- **5-element** system of Chinese acupuncture, translocation seems to dominate.
- **6-element** method suppression seems to dominate.
- **7-element** method transformation seems to dominate.
- **12-element** method both efficiency and transformation seem to dominate.
  - **As a STAR-model**
  - **As a 90^0-model**
- **Middle-point in a single patient**, the spiritual disease resolves but the physical pathology remains.
- **Middle-point in a circle** of patients, higher spiritual beings are enlisted and seem to help create a deeper and karmic spiritual healing among the entire group but physical pathology remains.

It is important to note the significance of *numerology* in treatment. I have come to realize that there is a strong correlation between the numbers of the paradigm and the spiritual structure of the society from which they emerged.

For example:
- the number four was emphasized by the Greeks, the society that embraced freedom as the elements of Water, Air, Earth and Fire.
- In contrast, the more patriarchal and class-structures of the Chinese adopted a more organized and controlled five element system which not only added the element wood but placed it in a generating and destructive sequence.
- The importance of a trinity was embraced by the Tibetans
- while the more sinister number six was emphasized by Jahvism and Islam, the merciless moon god.
- As an anthroposophist, I have found much interesting truth in the number seven, representing the work of Rudolf Steiner, which described the significance of this number in advancing the spiritual evolution of mankind.

- The number 12 mirrors the number of zodiacal signs, and as such encompass the whole of cosmos. It also expresses the number of the disciples around Jesus Christ, the truest transformational force known.

The choice of the system decided on will influence the results of our therapy, whether it will be a suppression, a translocation or a true transformation.

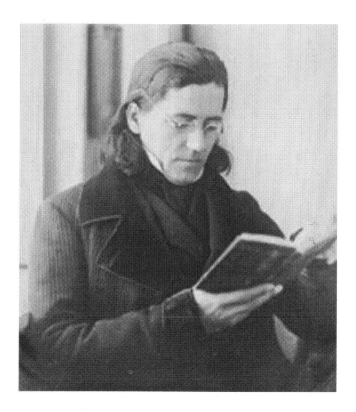

Constantine Hering M.D.

Learning through my fight on how to treat cancer.

Sometimes our greatest struggles guide us to our greatest achievements. For me, this struggle came with the treatment of cancer. The dilemma began with my use of acupuncture meridian therapy according to the five elements.[27]

My journey towards understanding the nature of cancer began in 1983. I realized at that time, cancer had to be treated differently from other disease processes. The solution seemed both simple and profound. Using the principles of five-element acupuncture, I saw cancer as simply an excess of a normal fundamental process. Therefore, the meridian organ system controlling that process must be deficient. My conclusion was to strengthen the deficient system and regain control over the excess. I called this method "the controlling treatment". I believed, at that time, that this was a superior treatment to directly treating the excess, which represented the western medical analogue of suppressing the growth of the tumors through surgery and chemotherapy. I was under the misguided belief that this might hold the key to curing cancer for the future.

For several years, the results seemed to prove my theory. In 1984, I first applied a "controlling" treatment method on a dachshund. The dog had multiple tumors along the mammary chain and was struggling to breath, indicative of pulmonary metastasis. Using acupuncture, I treated a strengthening point on the liver meridian (liver 03 – LR03), in order to tonify this meridian/organ system. As the liver controls the stomach meridian (the residence of the mammary chain) such a treatment should take control over the cancer. In a few weeks, the tumors disappeared completely. The dog died several years later from renal failure of old age.

Another example of this successful protocol occurred in 1995, when I used this method to treat my first horse cancer patient. The horse was diagnosed with an equine sarcoid, a form of skin cancer. The result was promising, as the sarcoid disappeared within six weeks.

---

[27] Holistic and spiritual veterinary medicine, Thoresen, Are, 2017. Amazon.

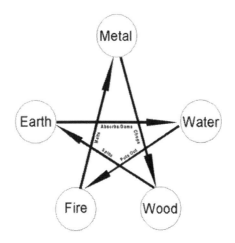

Between 1984 and 2014, I treated more than 1000 animal- and human-patients, suffering from all kinds of cancer. The results were especially good with mammary cancer (85%), and in melanoma (80%). The results in lymphosarcoma and brain cancer were moderately good (70%). However, my results with liver and pancreatic cancer were mediocre; the healing rate being "only" 60% in the few patients I treated.

My success with treating cancer patients using the 5-element controlling method continued for exactly 30 years up until 2014. I then *understood, intended and decided* to try to stop translocation. This mere willful *decision* triggered a huge response from the pathological entities. They sensed the looming disaster of transformation (demons seem to fear transformation). I began to notice a resistance to the five-element treatment. Although the tumors would still shrink, the actual ability to cure the patient declined. After some months the effect was totally gone. To make matters even more confusing, my closest students were experiencing the same phenomena. The only few that were still having some success where those physicians that had learned the method from my articles rather than directly through me. The efficacy of the controlling method on treating cancer continued to decline throughout 2014 until it was close to non-existent. I was baffled by this change in events.

I did not despair, but worked hard to find out the reason why the effect had vanished, and to find a better method.

The Middle-point, a new concept of treatment.

In 2016, I understood clearly that I could not use acupuncture according to the five-elements to treat cancer. I then decided to try employing the middle point. I discovered this point by studying the works of Judith von Halle[28].

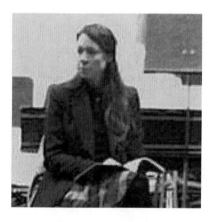

Judith von Halle (1972 -)

She stated that a diseased patient should be healed using "Christ-Consciousness".

I was still in confusion: how do I treat with a Christ consciousness?

---

[28] Judith von Halle was born 1972 in Berlin. She is an architect by profession and has worked as such. She has felt herself to be especially bound to Christ since childhood. She encountered anthroposophy in 1997 and worked part time for the German Anthroposophical Society until 2005. From 2001 till 2003 she gave lectures in the Rudolf Steiner House about esoteric Judaism and the Apocalypse of St. John. During Easter 2004 the stigmata of Christ appeared on her. Since that happened she has only been able to consume water – that is, no solid nourishment.

After looking carefully at the wooden sculpture called the Group or Representative of Man, made by Rudolf Steiner and Edith Maryon, depicting Christ standing between the two dominating adversary and pathological entities, Lucifer and Ahriman, I realized that the healthy energy of the Christ consciousness lies between these yin and yang structures residing in the body. I named the loci that could accomplish this task the "Middle Point". Using this point, I treat neither the excess nor the deficiency, but try to stimulate the middle or healthy area that lies between these two opposites.

The first time I attempted to treat the middle point was on a horse during a veterinary course in Germany. I clearly saw, with my spiritual eyes, a "Yin-pathological structure" (the ahrimanic double or demon) in the region of the abdomen, and a "Yang-pathological structure"" (the luciferic double or demon) in the region of the chest[29]. Using my spiritual vision, I could also locate the middle point.

I realized that these structures have a kind of "life force" of their own and, as such, require the gentler treatment of an acupuncture needle or even one's fingers. In contrast, a dermojet forces fluid into the point by a forceful thrust of pressurized air. Electrical stimulators, magnetic wave generators and cold lasers, are also ineffective and can be detrimental in treating the middle-point (the Christ point). This is due to the fact that the adversarial entities thrive off of these types of devices. Since 2014, I have treated many human and veterinary patients with the middle point, that is as single patients (and not in a group, as will be discussed later),

---

[29] The yang structures are almost always proximal or cranial. The yin structures are almost always distal or caudal. The Christ consciousness lies between them. In my book, spiritual medicine, this is discussed in detail

using one needle carefully placed in the middle, or with my fingers held in the gesture that Christ has in the group-statue made by Edith Maryon and Rudolf Steiner, **pushing the luciferic and the ahrimanic entities apart, making way for the Christ force to enter**. Most patients seem to be satisfied with the effect of this treatment, although the medical results seem to be less that the spiritual effect. This means that the healing takes place through the higher spiritual sheaths of the patient, and not directly through the etheric or physical body. Some patients describe an intense feeling of healing energy radiating throughout their bodies. I can see these patterns stream in the shape of a figure eight combined with a spiral.

I discovered that using the middle point seems to not heal the physical disease itself, but rather activates a more spiritual kind of healing. This is also the case when activating the middle-point in a group situation, that is treating several patients gathered together, sitting in a circle.

I also discovered that by combining the treatment of the middle with a non-translocating healing method (see later the 7-element method or especially the 12-element method), will initiate a curative response by healing both the material and the spiritual aspects of the patient.

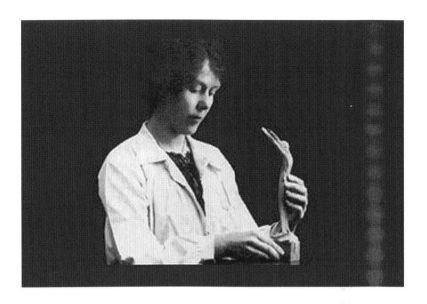

Edith Maryon (1872 – 1924)

The middle-point method transferred to 'classical' acupuncture (the acupuncture middle) explained through the 6-element method.

As most of my students were not able to spiritually visualize the middle point I hoped to find a way of combining the tools of pulse diagnosis, used in TCM (Traditional Chinese Medicine) to find a way for them to initiate Christ consciousness. I tried, with a suggestion from a colleague, to make two triangles out of the six pulses found on either side of the wrist. These pulses are used to find the pathological meridian processes of the patient. The triangles are shown below:

How to treat the middle after the 6 Principle

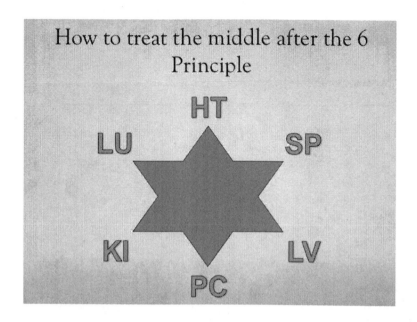

HT
LU   SP
KI   LV
PC

1. Left wrist: Heart (HT) – Kidney (KI) – Liver (LV).
2. Right wrist: Pericardium (PC) – Lung (LU) – Spleen (SP).

In these two triangles, I postulated that the middle should be the meridian that is between the excess and the deficiency as found by pulse diagnosis. If the main deficient pulse is on the left hand (either HT, LV or KI), let us say in this example that it is LV, we must then decide which of the other two pulses on this same wrist, HT or KI, is the relatively strongest. In this example we will assume it is the Kidney pulse. The Middle Point is then the remaining process, namely the HT. If the main deficiency is on the right hand, the middle will be either LU, SP or PC. Using this theory, one point is then needled on the meridian related to this Middle (Christ) Process.

However, after employing this technique I found it be ineffective and at times suppressive.

Acupuncture according to the "anatomical middle".

Another way of applying the principle of the middle to acupuncture is in the way of anatomy. In finding the excessive and the deficient areas on the body itself, we can treat the middle. It is just between the excess and the deficiency.

This middle can be found in three places:

- on the head (as in Cranio-Sacral therapy), expressing the Christ-force in thinking.
- at the chest, expressing the Christ-force in feeling.
- in the area of the abdomen, expressing the Christ-force in willing.

There are several ways to find this middle:

1.Seeing the middle point:(Clairvoyance)

The ability to "see" the spiritual world can be a natural gift or, with dedication, it can be learned. For me, it was a skill that I possessed since I was born. In my early youth it felt so natural that I assumed that everyone had this ability.

Although I use the word "see", this does not exactly convey the experience, as the physical eyes are not involved. For lack of a better description, this is as close a word I can use to describe the phenomenon. In order to gain access to the spiritual world, it is necessary to be able to excarnate from the material body as earlier explained.

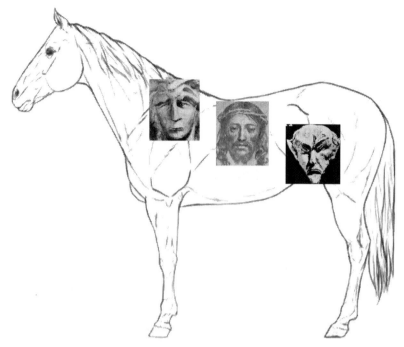

location of luciferic and ahrimanic demons in the body with Christ in the middle

2.Feeling the middle point (clairsentience).

This is the ability to receive information through sensing or feeling subtle energy. It is actually one of the more common psychic gifts often activated without conscious awareness. Loosely translated it means a "clear feeling". Clairsentience can trigger physical sensations such as tingling, a ringing in the ear, or changes in the practitioner's pulse. In extreme cases, one can even feel physical pain.

For some students, using Nogiér's pulse diagnosis to find the middle point is a form of effective clairsentience[30]. Nogiér, A French acupuncturist known for the development of auricular acupuncture, used the pulse as a kind of "Geiger counter" to find

---

[30] Auriculotherapy manual Chinese and western systems of ear acupuncture, Oleson, Terry, 2014, google books.

various pathologies. When a honing device was passed over a testing zone, the practitioner's pulse, taken at the auricular artery would change in rate or intensity. Using this same concept, one can pass the finger of one hand over the mid-section, while taking the auricular pulse with the other hand, and wait for a change in intensity or frequency.

Others have found that while performing this procedure, the patient often exhibits or experiences a change when the practitioner's finger is passed across the middle point. Horses are particularly sensitive and can be observed to chew, drop their heads and/or blink and close their eyes.

For many practitioners, the simple act of feeling the area can be informative. Some feel changes in temperature, while others feel a kind of roughness to the skin that, at a physical level, may not be overtly palpable.

3. Smelling the Middle Point:(Clairalience[31])

During the winter of 2017 I was teaching courses on how to find and treat the middle in both New York and Florida. In New York I had a student who claimed to have the ability to smell the presence of disease. With that proclamation, she insisted on smelling each patient to find the middle point, which she did accurately. I then proceeded to Florida to teach yet another group, and discovered that most did not possess the ability to spiritually 'see' the middle point. I decided then to test the efficacy of Clairalience. I began by emptying my lungs of air, and then with one long inhalation I passed my nostrils along the midsection of a canine patient. Much to my surprise, I found a clear change in the odor at the level of the midpoint. At the exact location, the odor changed from a normal dog smell to a more pleasant aroma.

---

[31] Clairalience: (Clair meaning "Clear" and "Alience" meaning scent) is the Psychic ability to be able to obtain specific Psychic information based on the use of the nose. Along with its sister abilities (Clairaudience, Clairvoyance, Claircognizance and Clairsentience), it makes up 5 of the 6 Psychic sense abilities.

Continuing beyond the point, however, revealed a pathological smell, quite distinct from the middle scent. After interviewing the course participants, I found that some were able to distinguish these three odors (normal – pathological – healing). I coined the phrase "the sniffing diagnostic test" for my new method of finding the middle point

The exact method involves exhaling all the air from the lungs, and with a long and constant inhalation through the nose move the head in a steady pace, over the back of the patient as shown below. To my surprise, I found it to be quite simple for me and several of the students to smell the middle point. At the exact Middle Point, the smell changes to a pleasant odor, and immediately cranial or caudal to the Middle, the smell changes to a somewhat more "physical", dog like, or even pathological smell. I asked the other participants to do this "sniffing-test", and about 60% of the participants could clearly recognize the 3 different smells.

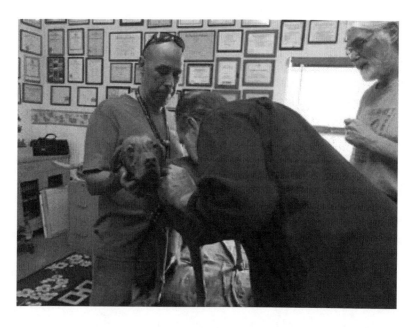

the "sniffing diagnostic test".

Using the Middle point in a transformative way to treat noxious earth radiation (as well as electromagnetic radiation, which will be discussed in chapter 6).

Earth-Radiation appears to my Spiritual eye, as black snakes curling and moving along the surface of the earth. They must not be mistaken for the energetic bonds between trees and plants, which are described in my book "Poplar". These bonds, although similar in their movement along the forest floor, are much lighter in hue. I have been able to enter these "tree snakes" with my consciousness, and as such, can travel within this energy pattern. Travelling in the left direction takes me back in time. I have never attempted to Travel to the right for fear of seeing the future. I consider the future belonging to higher powers than mine. Within the energetic streams of the trees, I have experienced the secret of the "double time stream".[32] The black snakes that are the expression of Earth-Radiation are 'seen' as darker and not as transparent as the tree energy snakes. Entering inside the earth-radiation snakes is not advisable, as they are of a malignant Ahrimanic nature. They represent the past deeds of all humans, the Karma of each of each and every one of us.

This Karma of past deeds can either be translocated or transformed, this choice is always ours to make.

- A *translocation* of the earth radiation can be achieved by applying a variety of technical devices, often based on ingenious systems of wires, metals and crystals. As these devices are made and exist in the material world, they usually just influence the material part of the radiation, while the real pathological element is the spiritual part - ahrimanic and/or luciferic elementals 'riding' the radiation.
- A *transformation* of earth radiation can be achieved by concentrating on the middle point within the earth

---

[32] **The double time stream** is one of the most important secrets we have to know about when entering the Spiritual world. Time can go either way, both from the future towards the past, and from the past against the future.

radiation itself as well as in the devises creating the electromagnetic radiation. By this concentration the strength of the Christ-force residing in the middle will be strengthened, and the adversarial forces will be pushed back, their cooperation weakened and hindered and finally (one may hope) transformed.

In healing and transforming both earth-radiation (which is created by human ill-deeds in this or in a former life) and electro-magnetic radiation (which is created or produced by binding and changing divine elementals, pushing them into under-nature, which is also a very ill deed), we should, as a fundamental mood in our soul when we deal with this kind of radiation, be asking forgiveness in the name of Christ.

Much the same procedure can be used to neutralize the pathological effect of EMR, and this will be dealt with further in chapter 6.

Using the Middle Point in a transformative way to treat plants and trees.

For many years I have been able to "pulse" trees. A German colleague, Ferdinand Niessen, told me he felt that all trees had a weakness in the water element about one third distal to the top of its structure. I pondered this phenomenon for years until I realized that all humans and animals have a deficiency of water where Lucifer abides, which is the top half of the body. As Lucifer represents heat, we often find a deficient kidney energy in that area. One third proximal to the root of the tree, and one third cranial to the tail base of animals and humans, we can find the Ahrimanic influence. Here there is a deficiency in the wood element, representing the energy and fundamental process of the liver as defined by Five Element Acupuncture. Therefore, when we pulse a tree, it is important that we do not pulse the tree 1/3 from the root or 1/3 from the top, otherwise we always get either a deficiency in the liver or in the kidney. In animals and humans this is the same. We have to focus and spiritually enter the heart of the patient to get a correct pulse finding. To treat a tree from the Middle-Point, we "needle it mentally" on the Middle Point between the kidney-deficiency and the liver-deficiency, and at the same time 'push' the adversaries back to make more room for the Christ-force. When I do this, I find that both the deficiencies often disappear.

Also, in treating trees this way we should hold within our souls, a feeling of asking for forgiveness in the name of Christ.

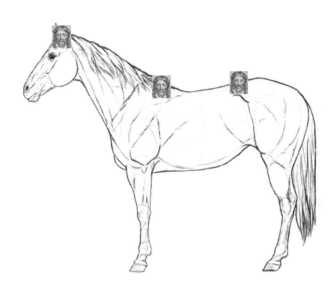

The 3 middle-points indicated by the presence of Christ

Using the middle-point in a circle of humans or animals.

On the evening of November 5th, 2016, something unexpected happened. I was giving a veterinary course in New York and decided to treat the participants with the middle point as a demonstration. Twenty-five human participants were lying on the floor as I needled all the individual midpoints between Lucifer and Ahriman. Then I sat back to watch. The needle that was placed on the thorax, between the adversaries, seemed to activate the area of "free" etheric force, not dominated by Ahriman or Lucifer; the Christ-force.

When this area became activated a light started to emanate from the chest of all the participants, and after a while it was rhythmically oscillating. After some time, the light started to float up from the participants and began to circle around and over the entire group. The circling became more and more luminous going upwards in a stream.

What I saw happening with the group was totally different from what happens when I treat an individual. The cooperation of the good in each and every one of the patients was able to transform something into light.

The irony of individualized treatment then became apparent. It was obvious that Ahrimanic forces are enhanced when man is "culled from the group". Sadly, the individualized approach to medical treatment has become the gold standard, especially with regards to immunotherapy. Without an understanding of spiritual science, the medical community is unaware of the power they are giving to the adversarial forces that perpetuate disease.

Rudolf Steiner predicted in the beginning of the 20th century, that mankind would become increasingly infused with technology. He also believed that this technology would be utilized by the adversaries to gain access and control over all aspects of human evolution. He was correct. Mechanization is another means by which ahrimanic forces can fortify their hold on the material world. Once again, it cannot be under stated that by using the social element of a group treatment, combined with the absence of machines, using only one single needle in the healthiest point of the body, namely the Christ point, can we go forward in preventing the disastrous cooperation between Lucifer and Ahriman.

Acupuncture according to 7 elements.

We have now seen that in using the 5-element treatment protocol we tend to *translocate* the pathology. In using the 6 elements we tend to *suppress* the pathology.

What if we now try to use the 7- or 12-elements? Here we will see that this works much more in a transformative way, especially the 12-element treatment, as did Christ work with transformation in his circle of 12 disciples.

Here I must make a short explanation about what 5-, 7- or 12 elements really mean. Man is a microcosm reflecting the great macrocosm. The Chinese observed in nature how the different elements worked together, and created the sequence of the 5 elements. The Greeks did the same with their 4 elements. We must then look to nature and see where we can find a seven-fold or 12-fold *structure*, with which we can create a nourishing cycle and a controlling cycle, the latter to be used in controlling cancer.

A possible solution through Anthroposophy: the 7-planetary 'elemental' system.

Many of us were introduced to biology by dissecting dead frogs, never learning anything about living frogs in nature. Modern biology has moved out of nature and into the laboratory, driven by a desire to find an underlying mechanistic basis of life. Despite all its success, this approach is one-sided and urgently calls for a counterbalancing movement toward nature. Only if we find ways of transforming our tendency to reduce the world to parts and mechanisms, will we be able to see, value, and protect the integrity of nature and the interconnectedness of all things. This demands a new way of seeing. Anthroposophy is a spiritual science inspired by integrative thinkers and scientists, such as Johann Wolfgang von Goethe, Rudolf Steiner and Kurt Goldstein. This philosophy allows us to develop ways of perception that integrate self-reflective and critical thought, imagination, and careful, detailed observation of the phenomena of nature.

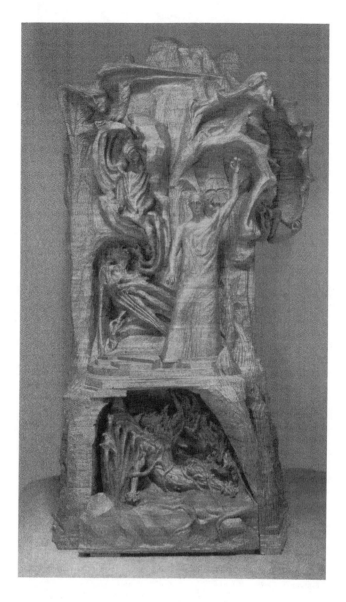

Christ in the middle between Lucifer and Ahriman

According to these principles, the organism teaches us about itself, revealing its characteristics and its interconnectedness with the world that sustains it. This way of doing science enhances our sense of responsibility for nature. As Goethe states, all of nature's individual aspects are interconnected and interdependent. All the parts of an individual have a direct effect on one another, a relationship between one another, thereby constantly renewing the circle of life. Thus, we are justified in considering every animal physiologically perfect. By understanding these tenants, I finally understood that I had to transform the **perceptions** of a pre-Christian system (the law of the five elements) to a post-Christian system, based on anthroposophy. Maybe I could use the Goetheanistic observations of the cosmos and its inhabitants that anthroposophy is so known for?

The most important and fundamental concept in anthroposophy is the 7-fold division of time and of space. I theorized that it would be possible to make two new systems, one based on the 7-foldness of space, and one based on the 7-foldness of time.

Finding the 7-fold system of space (heliocentric and geocentric system).

We relate the spatial relationship of the 7 planets to the 7 organ-meridian processes of Traditional Chinese Medicine. These relationships are recorded in several ancient texts and are shown below;

- Sun: Heart (HT)
- Moon: Reproductive organs (PC)
- Mercury: Intestines, lung (LU, LI, SI)
- Venus: Kidney (KI)
- Mars: Gallbladder (GB)
- Jupiter: Liver (LR or LV)
- Saturn: Spleen (SP)

This represents a total of 7 planets and 7 organ-meridian systems instead of the 5 or 6 organ-meridian systems dealt with by the Chinese. I was then faced with the problem of how to arrange these 7 planets and organs to find the controlling and nourishing sequence as used in the five-element system. After much trial and error, I came down with four possible ways, which I tried to combine in my therapy for two years before I found the 12-element system which now seems to be the most effective, and which also can be combined with the middle point, either individually or in a group.

1. Arrange the 7 elements according to space in the heliocentric system.
2. Arrange the 7 elements according to space in the geocentric system.
3. Arrange the 7 elements according to time in a 7-point star-structure.
4. Arrange the 7 elements according to time in a cradle structure (phasic evolution of the cosmos according to

Steiner) i.e.: the downward phase is a mirror of the upward phase.

The Anthroposophic 7 organ-processes in space.

Method 1: The heliocentric system (Processes as the planets are ordered as seen from the sun).

In this system:

- Heart controls Kidney yang (Reproductive organs).
- Kidney yin (the kidney organ itself) controls Liver.
- Gall-bladder controls Heart.
- Lung controls Gall-Bladder.
- Liver controls Lung and Intestines.
- Kidney yang (Reproductive organs) controls Spleen.
- Spleen controls Kidney.

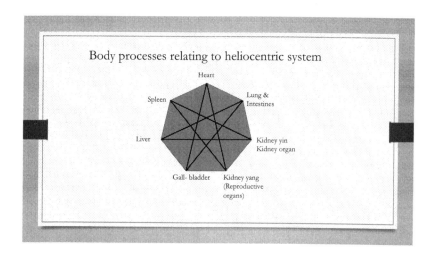

Body processes relating to heliocentric system

Method 2: The geocentric system (Processes as the planets are ordered as seen from the earth).

In this system:

- Heart controls Spleen.
- Kidney (yin) controls Heart.
- Gall-bladder controls Kidney yin (Kidney).
- Lung (and intestines) controls Gall-bladder.
- Liver controls Lung and intestines.
- Kidney yang (reproductive parts) controls Liver.
- Spleen controls Kidney yang (the adrenals).

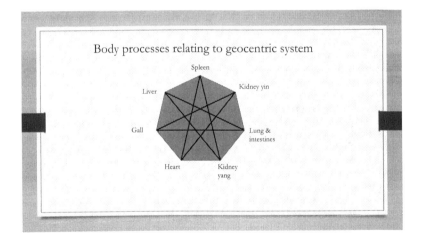

Method 3: Using the order of the planets according to the development of our planetary system, as described by Rudolf Steiner.

In this system:

- Spleen controls Gall-bladder.
- Kidney controls Liver.
- Gall-bladder controls Reproduction (Pericardium).
- Lung controls Spleen.
- Liver controls Heart.
- Pericardium controls Kidney
- Spleen controls Gall-bladder

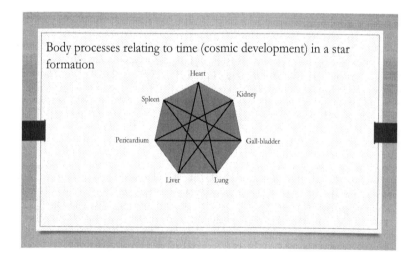

The 12-element zodiacal system.

Method 4: The zodiacal system as viewed as a star (Order of the processes as the zodiacal constellations are arranged in the cosmos).

Where:

- Spleen controls Liver.
- Small Intestine controls Stomach.
- Bladder controls Heart.
- Large Intestine controls Kidney.
- Trippel Heater controls Lung.
- Liver controls Pericardium.
- Stomach controls Gall-bladder.
- Heart controls Spleen.
- Kidney controls Small Intestine.
- Lung controls Bladder.
- Pericardium controls Large Intestine.
- Gall Bladder controls Trippel Heater.

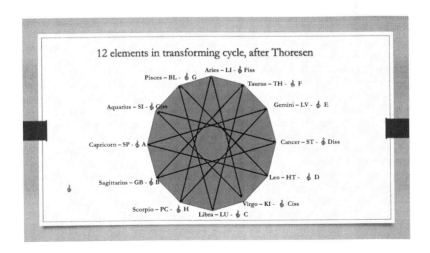

This system I have now used since December 2018, on >1000 patients of all types. The results have been the best I have ever seen, with strong effects and transforming results.

I have not yet had time to make statistics on the effects and results according to the different diseases, but this will be done in the near future.

This system is used like the other systems. If the problem, both the deficiency or the excess, for example is in the liver (LV), then treat this problem with the ting-point of the spleen (SP).[33]

---

[33] Thinking must be used in the initial stage of the diagnosis of any patient, both animal and man. We must inquire about the nature of the disease, make our observations and determine how to perform the treatment. Is surgery needed, is the horse dangerous, can the dog bite us, do we need any medications and so on?

Then we proceed to the method of separating Thinking, Feeling and Willing as described in this book. When we have reached this state of mind, we proceed to focus on the soul faculty of Feeling, visualizing the heart. Here is when we leave the thinking and willing behind. We imagine spiritually entering the 12th layer of the heart of the patient. We imagine a tunnel from our heart to the heart of the patient. This tunnel traverses all 12 layers of the body coming to an end at the center of the patient's heart.

Keeping our focus here, we make our diagnosis. Personally, I use the pulse-diagnosis to go through all the different processes of the body, both in the present time and in the past, however any modality of Spiritual diagnosis may be used whether it be homeopathy, kinesiology or any method that may give the information we need. We can also go into the processes of the forefathers and foremothers, investigating the different physical, mental or spiritual traumas. In doing this, we mentally organize the information that we have gathered. This is when we combine the Thinking with the Feeling.

When we have decided with our Thinking how to treat the disease, we leave both the thinking and the feeling behind, and enter into the Will power of the universe, which is to be found in the earth itself. This Will force must be used in the therapeutic part of the procedure. The focus of the therapist will then be in his limbs, his feet, or even in the earth beneath his feet. From this area, the force of the Will is awakened, and this force will then stream up through the body. The path this force takes is not along the spine, described as the "Kundalini" force in old traditions. This up-going stream should be found in front of the spine. The force in the spine is of the old world, related to Lucifer. The force of the new world is in the middle of the body, related to Christ. It is possible to experience this up-going stream as a dance between two snakes,

The appearance of the 3 double-crosses in the 12-element controlling circle. A possible transition from pre- to post-Christian thinking.

If we look carefully on the structure of the 12-star, we will soon realize an interesting geometric pattern. The structure actually consists of 3 crosses, each formed as a double-cross.

The first cross consists of the axis of the BL to LI and LU to KI, crossed with the horizontal axis of SP to GB and LV to ST. All the diagonals in this cross are acupuncture Yin-Yang pairs.

The second cross consists of the axis of the SI to the BL and the KI to the HT, crossed with the horizontal axis of GB to PC and TH to LV. All the diagonals in this cross are within acupuncture Yin-Yang pairs.

The third cross consists of the axis SP-SI and HT-ST, crossed with the horizontal axis of PC-LU and LI-TH. All the diagonals in this third cross are again within acupuncture Yin-Yang pairs.

---

one white and one black. This force must then enter the heart and mingle with the feeling, compassion and love for the patient, and, in fact, for the whole of humanity. If we activate the Kundalini force, this goes straight to the crown chakra, and does not stop at the level of the heart. This mingling often results in a feeling of Cosmic divine love, inhabiting the center of the heart. From this center, the healing force, now totally cleaned from any egoistic wish or intent, streams over into the patient. Here, directed by intentional thought that streams down from the head, the healing force works in the body by diminishing the power of the Demons. If this force is directed against the ahrimanic demon, the healing of the organic structures will begin. If it is directed against the luciferic demon, the pain and unpleasantness will diminish. If it is directed to the Middle, the Christ-Point or the Christ-filled gap between the two Demons, both Demons will pull back and start to dissolve or Transform.

The KVINT-circle and the countercurrent CROMATIC circle that appear in the 12-element zodiacal transformative circle.

I have for many years studied the relationship between the 12 tones in our scale and the zodiacal constellations.

Likewise, I have also studied the relationship between the acupuncture meridians and the musical tones.

- There are 12 meridians
- There are 12 zodiacal signs
- There are 12 tones in our music

When we have arranged in a circle as showed above, the zodiacal signs as a continuous succession, just as in the cosmos, we get the succession as follows, starting with Libra: Libra - Scorpio - Sagittarius - Capricorn - Aquarius - Pisces - Aries - Taurus - Gemini - Cancer - Leo - Virgo.

If we then add the relating meridians to this succession we get the following line: LU - PC - GB - SP - SI - BL - LI - TH - LV - ST - HT - KI.

We also see from the figure of the 12 signs that the controlling functions (the lines in the star-formation) are related to the KVINT, as the succession of musical tones are as follows: C - H - B - A - Giss - G - Fiss - F - E - Diss - D - Ciss.

For example, we see that as LU is controlling BL, then the related tones will be C and G, which constitutes a KVINT. And so it is with all the meridians and tones.

Also, it is worthwhile to observe that if we follow the notes counterclockwise, we get the CROMATIC scale of C - Ciss - D - Diss - E - F - Fiss - G - Giss - A - B - H and again C.

The appearance of the 3 single-crosses in the 12-element controlling circle. A possible description of the power-flow of the universe.

If we look carefully at the structure of the 12-star, we will soon begin to realize an even more interesting geometric pattern. The structure actually consists of 3 single crosses, each expressing the power-constellations of the cosmos.

1. The first cross consists of the axis of the BL to KI, crossed with the horizontal axis of LV to GB. This cross relates, according to Rudolf Steiner, to the morning – evening – axis of Christ (Pisces) and Sophia (Virgo), which are positive forces. This axis is then crossed by the diagonal of midday – midnight, of Ahriman (Gemini) and Lucifer (Sagittarius), which are evil forces.
2. The second cross consisting of the axis of the LI to LU, being crossed by SP to ST.
3. The third cross consists of the axis of the TH to PC, being crossed by SI to HT.

These relations offer us another insight into a controlling and transforming therapy, which will be explained after the following quotation of Rudolf Steiner.

If we take a closer look at the **spiritual forces** emanating from the different constellations, we find Steiners words[34] somewhat enlightening:

---

[34] «Reappearance of Christ in the Etheric", lecture 12, held on the 25th of November 1917, by Rudolf Steiner, GA 178.

And so, just as it is essential for an orthodox professor of biology to have the most powerful microscope available and the most efficient laboratory methods, so, in the future, when science has been spiritualized, it will be of the utmost importance whether certain processes are carried through in the morning or in the evening, or at midday, and whether what has been done in the morning is allowed to be further influenced by an evening activity, or whether the cosmic influences are cut out, paralyzed, from the morning until the evening. Processes of this kind will of necessity come to light and will run their course. Naturally, a great deal of water will have to flow under the bridges before the professional chairs and laboratories, at present organized on purely materialistic lines, are handed over to spiritual scientists, but this replacement must come about if humanity is not to sink into utter decadence. For example, if the question is one of doing good in the immediate future, existing laboratory methods must give way to methods whereby certain processes take place in the morning and are interrupted during the day, so that the cosmic stream passes through them again in the evening and is in turn rhythmically withheld again until morning. So, the processes would take their course: certain cosmic workings would always be interrupted by day, and the cosmic morning and evening processes would be brought in. All sorts of arrangements would be necessary for this. You will realize that if one is not in a position to take any public action about these things, all one can do is to speak of them.

However, just as gold, health and the prolongation of life are put in the place of God, virtue and immortality, so from the same quarter efforts will be made to work not with the morning and evening processes, but with others.

Last week I told you how an attempt will be made to set aside the impulse of the Mystery of Golgotha, while for the West another impulse, a sort of Antichrist is introduced; and from the East an attempt will be made to paralyze the twentieth century manifestation of the Christ Impulse by diverting attention from the coming etheric Christ.

Those concerned to present an Anti-Christ as the real Christ will try also to make use of something that works through the most material forces, but in this very way can work spiritually. Above all they will strive to make use of electricity and earth-magnetism in order to produce effects all over the world. I have shown you how earth-forces rise up into what I have called the human Double, the Doppelgänger. This secret will be opened up. An American secret will be to make use of earth-magnetism, with its north-south duality, and by this means to send over the earth guiding forces which will have spiritual effects. Look at the magnetic chart of the earth and compare it with what I am now saying. Observe where the magnetic needle deviates to East and West and where it does not deviate. I can give only hints about all this. From a certain direction in the heavens, spiritual beings are continually active, and they have only to be put into the service of the earth, and — because these beings working in from the cosmos can mediate the secret of the earth's magnetism — it will be possible for egotistic groups to get behind this secret and to accomplish a great deal in connection with gold, health and the prolongation of life. It will be necessary for them only to pluck up their faltering courage — and in certain circles that will be done readily enough!

From the East an endeavor will be made to strengthen what I have already explained: to place in the service of the earth the beings which work in from the opposite side of the cosmos. In the future there will be a great battle. Human science will stretch out to the cosmic, but will try to get there by different paths. It will be the task of good, healing science to find certain cosmic forces which can reach the earth through the co-operation of two cosmic streams, those of Pisces and Virgo. The great secret to be discovered will be how the influence which works from the direction of Pisces as a power of the sun unites itself with the influence working from the direction of Virgo. It will make for good when it is learnt how the morning and evening forces from the two sides of the cosmos can be brought into the service of humanity.

These forces, however, will be left aside by those who try to achieve their whole purpose through the polaric duality of positive and negative forces. The forces which enable the spiritual to stream down to earth with the aid of positive and negative magnetism come from Gemini; they are the midday forces. In ancient times it was known that cosmic influences were involved in this, and to-day even exoteric scientists are aware that in some or other way positive and negative magnetism lie behind Gemini in the Zodiac. The aim will be to paralyze all that could be gained through a revelation of the true duality in the cosmos — to paralyze it in a materialistic, egotistic way by means of the forces which stream in particularly from Gemini and can be placed entirely at the service of the human "Double."

Other brotherhoods, concerned above all to divert attention from the Mystery of Golgotha, will try to make use of the duality in human nature — the duality which in our epoch embraces man as a unity, but includes within him his lower animal nature. A human being is really a centaur in a certain sense: his humanity rests on his lower *animal nature in its astral form. This working together of the duality in man gives rise to a duality of forces. This duality of forces will be utilized particularly by certain egotistic brotherhoods, chiefly from the side of India and the East, in order to mislead eastern Europe, whose task it is to prepare for the sixth post-Atlantean epoch. And this will be done with the aid of the forces which work in from Sagittarius.*

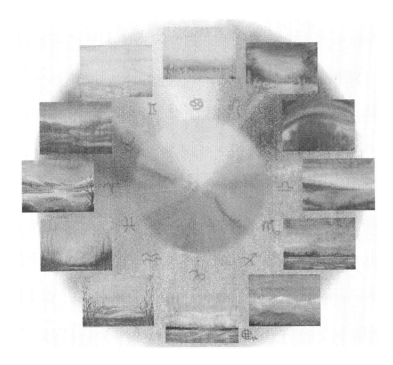

Be aware of the three single crosses.

Our 'logical' conception of reality in making everything into polarities is for me like being dragged into Maya, as I consider the middle to be the only force of reality, our only salvation.

The polarities seem to me to be an expression of the great illusion, whilst the trinity expresses the reality.

It is of vital importance to find this third aspect in all uses of electricity, magnetism, nuclear power, cosmic streams or corporeal balances, otherwise the ahrimanic-luciferic forces will dominate.

We find the same opposition between duality and trinity in the soul forces of thinking, feeling and willing. Within each we must find the middle point, the middle force, and if we can then relate to and use this middle, this force of LOVE as a fourth force permeating the cosmos, we have a cross, similar to the morning-evening-midday-midnight forces.

The only salvation is to add the force of LOVE to the fundamental forces.

That is why the symbol reflecting the love of Jesus Christ is a CROSS.

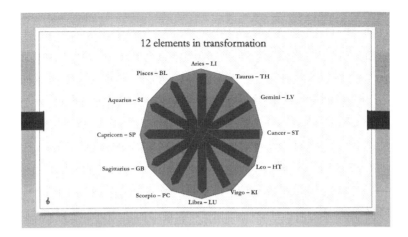

12 elements in transformation

How the middle can heal the adversarial forces.

Here we see a picture of the main opposing forces represented by the line between Pisces and Virgo and the opposing or adversary forces exposing themselves in the line between Sagittarius and Gemini.

The interesting observation is that the healing forces from Pisces (Christ) can transform the forces of Gemini (Ahriman), and the healing forces of Virgo (Sophia) can heal the adversarial forces of Sagittarius (Lucifer), and that these healing forces arrive in a 90^0 (degree) angel.

The next two pages illustrate how this healing force can be extended to cover all the different constellations, bearing in mind that the healing forces always arrive in a 90^0 (degree) angel.

Here we see how this healing force can be active through the whole circle of organs or stellar forces.

The 12-element zodiacal system.

Method 5: The zodiacal system as viewed as a quadratum (in a 90⁰ angel) (Order of processes as the constellations are ordered in the cosmos).

Where in this system:

- Gall-bladder heals Bladder (in a Christ/Sophia-like way).
- Liver heals Kidney (in a Christ/Sophia-like way).
- Spleen heals Large Intestine (in a Christ/Sophia-like way).
- Small Intestine heals hormonal system (in a Christ/Sophia-like way).
- Bladder heals Liver (in a Christ/Sophia-like way).
- Large Intestine heals Stomach (in a Christ/Sophia-like way).
- hormonal system heals Heart (in a Christ/Sophia-like way).
- Liver heals Kidney (in a Christ/Sophia-like way).
- Stomach heals Lung (in a Christ/Sophia-like way).
- Heart heals Pericardium (in a Christ/Sophia-like way).
- Kidney heals Gall bladder (in a Christ/Sophia-like way).
- Lung heals Spleen (in a Christ/Sophia-like way).

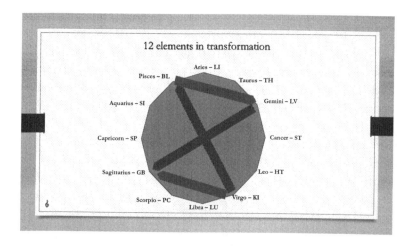

In this system we have 3 quadrats:

1. Hormonal system – Heart – Pericardium – Small Intestine.
   This is the feeling-inter(by love)-healing-system.
2. Liver – Kidney – Gall bladder – Bladder.
   This is the willing-inter(by love)-healing-system.
3. Stomach – Lung – Spleen – Large intestine.
   This is the thinking-inter(by love)-healing-system.

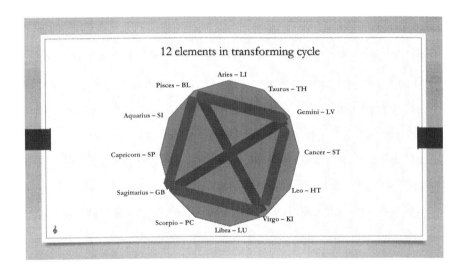

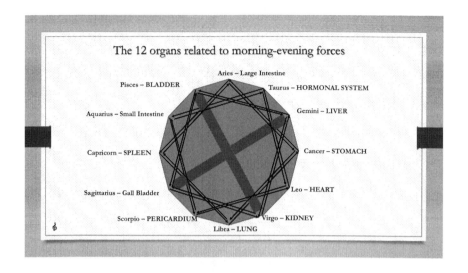

The 12 organs related to morning-evening forces

Aries – Large Intestine
Pisces – BLADDER
Taurus – HORMONAL SYSTEM
Aquarius – Small Intestine
Gemini – LIVER
Capricorn – SPLEEN
Cancer – STOMACH
Sagittarius – Gall Bladder
Leo – HEART
Scorpio – PERICARDIUM
Virgo – KIDNEY
Libra – LUNG

Where in this system:

- Liver and Gall-bladder heals Kidney and Bladder (in a Christ/Sophia-like way).
- Kidney and Bladder heals Liver and gall-bladder (in a Christ/Sophia-like way).
- Heart and Small Intestine heals Pericardium and Trippel Heather (in a Christ/Sophia-like way).
- Pericardium and Trippel Heather heals Heart and Small Intestine (in a Christ/Sophia-like way).
- Lung and Large Intestine heals Spleen and Stomach (in a Christ/Sophia-like way).
- Spleen and Stomach heals Lung and Large Intestine (in a Christ/Sophia-like way).

An explanation to the last figure.
Here, in this last figure we see how the masculine and feminine forces together can heal.

First, we had separated the masculine and the feminine from the 5-elemets to a 12 element-cycle, where the masculine and the feminine had been separated, and then, as shown in the last figure, both the masculine and the feminine can work together in healing the disease.

In this way liver and gall bladder can together heal both the kidney and the bladder.

In this way we will have:

1. Liver and Gallbladder together heals Kidney and Bladder and vica versa.
2. Lung and large Intestine together heals Spleen and Stomach and vica versa.
3. Heart and Small intestine together heals pericardium and Hormonal system and vica versa.

In this way man and woman, Christ and Sophia, join their forces in healing the world.

Salvatore Mundi.

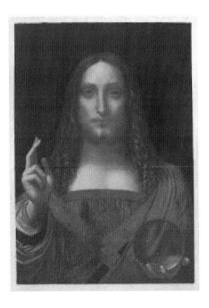

The dangers of the 5-element model.

Written by Dr. Margaret Mary Fleming, DVM, AP

The Wu Xing

The fundamental question after the sudden failure of his five-element approach was, "why did it happen?". As stated previously, he found his first clue in the advice of Judith von Halle, to find a way that employs the Christ impulse. However, those not versed in the philosophy of anthroposophy might wonder why the absence of such thinking would cause such a time-honored tradition as Traditional Chinese Medicine and its theory of the five elements to fail in such a monumental way? The answers often lie in the past, in the understanding of the nature of the origin of these concepts well before they were distorted and eroded with time.

The pin yin for five elements is Wu Xing which can also be interpreted as the five phases, the five movements or the five planets (Jupiter, Saturn, Mercury, Venus, and Mars) (Mark that the sun is not included!!!). The word phase is superior to element, which was a word that was transposed from Greek culture which observed natural physical phenomena as divided into the four elemental categories of Earth, Fire, Air, and Water. The fifth element of Chinese thought is wood, which represents the planet of Jupiter and the dynamic function of the liver in developing will power and allowing our destiny to unfold. This is interesting with regards to anthroposophy, as Jupiter shall be the next evolutionary phase when the Earth phase is completed. It also worthwhile to note that Manfred Porkert, a prominent authority on the subject, wrote that the best meaning he had found for this symbol was a series of evolutionary phases, but this term was discarded due to its length. However, he expanded on this idea when he defined these evolutionary phases as dynamic "interdependent" aspects of the development of the universe. However, over time, these five phases have been distorted to represent almost all aspects of Chinese material life.

The first mention of the five elements extended as far back as the earliest records of Chinese history nearly 3000 years ago. At that time, it was stated that it is a way to describe natural processes that were hidden from our view. A definition rather reminiscent of the spiritual world. A text from the Zuo Zhuan refers to the elements as being formed by "officials" that are presented as spirits or deities which require offerings to be made to them. The Tibetan religion, Bon, also embraced the five-element philosophy, but referred to the phases as experiential sensations of the natural world. According to this religion, the elemental processes are fundamental metaphors for working with external, internal, and secret energetic forces and believe they are all aspects of a primordial energy. It is also stated in their scriptures that the five elements reflect successive phases in our becoming human beings. Throughout these phases our experience is reflected as God like with intensities of illumination and with each element having a distinct bright color of light.

As time passed the spiritual connotations of the five elements as a way to respect the universe and the order of things as an upright moral being were minimized, and the emphasis was placed on it as a medical system. This occurred in the Han dynasty when Daoist notions of immortality were professed.

By the first century B.C. the Huangdi Neijing (The yellow Emperors Inner Classic) became the premier textbook regarding Huang-Lao (Yellow emperor Laozi) Daoism. In this work, the subject of acupuncture and Chinese Medicine is elaborated. The emphasis is placed on the concept of the body being a microcosm of the universe.

The Yellow God (Huang Di)

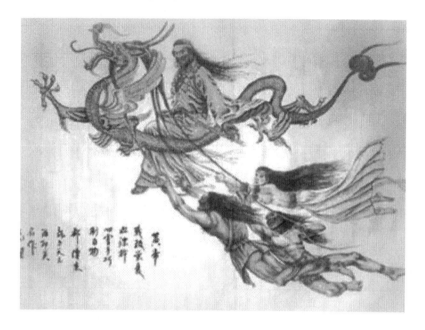

"Why are there no more Dragons?"

-The Duke of Zhao   600 BC

The Yellow Emperor appeared in the ancient texts approximately 2700 B.C. who most scholars agree, was first described as the "God of Light". Historians claim he was derived from Shang Di, who was considered the highest God of the Shang Dynasty. In addition, according to Sarah Allen, an expert on this subject, he was originally an unnamed being referred to as "the Lord of the Underworld" and was depicted as a dragon. His mother, Fubao, was a virgin who, through an immaculate conception conceived him after being hit by a lightning bolt. To continue the thread that he was perceived as a spiritual being, folklore has recounted an event when he visited the mythical east sea and met a talking beast. This beast taught him the knowledge of all supernatural creatures. Also called the "Yellow Deity with Four Faces" he represents the center of the universe and by regulating the heart within, he brings order without. It was also written that he said in order to reign one must reduce himself abandoning emotions. Similar to Steiner's concept of the separation of thinking, feeling, and willing, Huang Di went out into the wilderness to Mt. Bowang in order to find himself. It was said at this point that he created a void where the forces of creation gathered that made him more powerful. He imparted the concept that the center (similar to the middle) is also the vital point in the microcosm that is man, and that this center is where the internal universe is described as an altar. He further elaborated on the idea that the body is a universe and that by going into himself and incorporating the structure of the universe, he will gain access to the gates of heaven. Finally, he is also seen as a manifestation of the divine order encased in a physical reality that will open to immortality. These statements that have been made, reflect similarities to the life of Jesus as in incarnation of Christ. Complete with a virgin birth, a temptation in the wilderness and the promise of eternal life. Thus, the implication is that he is a reincarnation of a higher spiritual being. But what being could he be?

The Incarnation of Lucifer.
Steiner delivered a lecture on November 15th, 1919 in the town of Dornach Switzerland, home of the center of anthroposophy. There he told the story of three of the most important incarnations of high spiritual beings that have and will shape the destiny of all of mankind. How we develop as selfless spiritual beings, and how we cope with the lessons, gifts, and challenges that these three powerful figures bestow upon us will determine the fate of humanity. These three spiritual beings are none other than Lucifer, Christ, and Ahriman.

Steiner recounts the beginning of our evolution by reminding us that our human soul contained, from the beginning, a powerful primeval wisdom. But in the beginning the seed of this wisdom had to be nurtured to achieve the spiritual heights we needed to attain to become developed beings in a material existence. We needed a spiritual guide from the higher hierarchies to assist us in the growth of our I consciousness. This teacher was the descended archangel called Lucifer. The time of his incarnation onto Earth was estimated by Rudolf Steiner to be around 3000 BC and the setting was in the east in the Asian region. In the previous paragraphs, we have researched the ancient archives regarding the story of the Yellow emperor named Huang Di and have shown that his appearance occurred at the same time and in the same location. It is thus logical to assume that the body that received the incarnation of the light bearer was none other than this yellow deity. For those of us practicing the ancient art of Traditional Chinese Medicine, particularly five-element acupuncture, this historical correlation is of paramount importance. This might be the first clue why Are Thoresen's five element cancer protocol became not only ineffective, but may have never been a truly transformational approach. It appears that these concepts that employ a luciferic impulse, despite their alluring nature, are ultimately outdated and even dangerous tools. They must now be replaced by a higher impulse that came 3000 years later with the advent of the second incarnation, that of Christ.

Lucifer, as Huang Di, brought us the world of thought and speech, the characteristics necessary to develop our "I" through a pagan wisdom. This wisdom could be only obtained from luciferic sources and the initiates of the time were obligated to receive it without becoming tainted by the ulterior motives of the light bearer, which is to abandon the path of earth evolution, to win mankind for a kingdom alien to that of Christ. As has been stated earlier, the gifts of Lucifer are a unification of man, spiritual inspiration and creativity. After all, Lucifer is leading us with the brighter light away from our intended path. However, the lure of material and separationism is always there to swing our consciousness toward the other side of the pendulum, leading to a disdain of the spiritual with a kind of stark rigidity and toward the world of the third future incarnation, that of Ahriman. According to Steiner, he shall incarnate in the west 3000 years after the incarnation of Christ.

The tendency to split up into groups and to form different nations and different languages creating greed and dissent gave fodder for the development of an ahrimanic impulse. This impulse is characterized by a hatred of spiritual science and the ease of being simply given a kind of false gift of clairvoyance in the future. Without a counterbalance, mankind will succumb to his rigid, cold and ossified kingdom on earth with no hope for complete spiritual evolution. This counterbalance, employing the Christ impulse, must be nurtured now during this epoch. In this way, Christ will be able to stand between the two adversaries who can bestow their positive traits to our education and advancement, but be kept at bay by the power of Christ standing in the middle. Therefore, it is our responsibility, as it is of all of mankind, to not allow Ahriman to consume us with materialism.

Steiner felt that the main tool to combat Ahriman is the philosophy of spiritual science. In addition, any luciferic methodology will create a bypass around Christ allowing both adversaries to join hands and destroy all hope for our spiritual redemption. Thus, our task is to focus all our efforts toward employing those tools that facilitate the evolution of man toward reunification with the Saturn primal energy and to eventually become part of the hierarchy of spiritual beings. Real wisdom has to be obtained not from ahrimanic complacency, but from the struggle of sacrifice and pain. For in this struggle, we prevent the rigidification of our world and allow the warmth of the Christ impulse to return to infuse future Vulcan. Therefore, humans are balanced between Lucifer and Ahriman and Christ is our wingman leading us away from the ending battle with Lucifer to engage in the future battle against Ahriman

Finally, in regard to treatment, Steiner discusses the importance of numerology in this equation. He felt that the old pagan ways were reflected in the pentagon and the number five, which is considered a symbol for Lucifer. Therefore, when we engage the five-element system in treatment, we are actually strengthening Lucifer and counteracting the Christ impulse. The hexagon, however, reflects the number six, symbolizing the power of Ahriman. Therefore, using the hexagon in acupuncture, for example, fast forwards us to the world of Ahriman. The number reflecting our spiritual evolution, however, is achieved by the use of the number seven, reflected in the 7 planetary phases, the seven passions of the Christ, and the newly formed treatment protocols using the 7-e system.

The incarnation of Christ 3000 years after the incarnation of Lucifer gave humanity something of immense brilliance. The Christ impulse returned our primeval wisdom which was taken up by the hearts and minds of the best of us, that is, the citizens of a civilized society. What we must do to prevent our captivity by Ahriman is to:

- understand and appreciate the materialistic world of mathematics and mechanistic laws, but appreciate that ultimately these are illusions. We must never lose sight of the reality of a spiritual world.
- The second thing we must do is to work toward joining hands in selfless love with one another in peace and harmony.
- And finally, by understanding that Ahriman gains a foot hold by dividing and conquering, we must emphasize the importance and power of group therapy in acupuncture, group meditation in communities, and group love for all.

To be able to diagnose disease spiritually we have to enter the spiritual world.

Traditional Chinese Medicine and The Pulse.

How to train to do something in the spiritual world concerning transformation and translocation.

Our third tool.

Traditional Chinese Medicine and The Pulse.
The aspect of pulse diagnosis as part of an acupuncture protocol is complex. Over thousands of years, it has undergone a metamorphosis as a result of a division in TCM between two often fundamentally opposed concepts:

- The first concept revolves around what is termed the *eight-principle theory*.
- The other field of TCM that has evolved from a completely different construct is termed *five-element acupuncture*.

In *eight-principle theory* the principles are bipolar in nature (*not trinitarian !!!*) and are guided by what the physician will prescribe as an herbal formula. The patient is evaluated based on the following eight criteria:

1. Is the global picture of the patient Yin? (interior, cold, deficient)
2. Is the global picture of the patient Yang? (exterior, hot, excess)
3. Is the disease deeply imbedded and chronic (interior)?
4. Is the disease superficial and acute (exterior)?
5. Is the disease one of excess?
6. Is the disease one of deficiency?
7. Is the disease cold?
8. Is the disease hot?

The physician then uses the *four examinations* (listening, looking, touching, and smelling) to determine an appropriate herbal protocol to address the findings.

The examination that we shall focus on is that of touch, of which taking the pulse plays a pivotal role. In addition to finding the answer to the above eight questions, the pulse can also help us determine the nature of what TCM calls the *4 fundamental substances* critical to the functioning of the organism:

1. The fundamental substance of Yin (estrogen).
2. The fundamental substance of Yang (thyroxin).
3. The fundamental substance of Blood (RBC s).
4. The fundamental substance of Fluid (joint fluid).

In order to take the pulse, the physician places his fingers on the radial artery of the patient's left and right wrist. Depicted below is the position of where the pulse is taken. Note that the pulses on each wrist have a positional dependence, as each of the practitioner's second third and fourth finger can access the health of a specific meridian-organ.

In addition, the pulse will reveal several global aspects of the patient. In this case, the practitioner will check if the pulse is rapid (heat) or slow (cold), strong in force verses only slightly perceptible (excess vs deficiency), and more subjective qualities that denote specific organ involvement. This would include a wiry quality (as if you were feeling a guitar string) of a liver imbalance or the rolling action of a spleen imbalance likened to a wave under your finger. With this information, the diagnostician prepares a formula that would address these abnormal characteristics.

The other field of TCM that has evolved from a completely different construct is termed *five-element acupuncture*. This field of knowledge is based more on the aspects of selecting acupuncture points to balance the patient rather than the administration of herbal concoctions. Basically, the organ meridian processes are placed in categories analogous to the elements found in nature listed as Fire, Earth, Metal, Water and Wood. This form of acupuncture also requires feeling the pulse at the radial arteries of the wrists, but pays much more attention to the *relative* strength of each position of the pulse along the length of that artery. The practitioner concerns himself more with where the weakest pulse is found and how it compares to the other organ/meridians that are being accessed. This latter technique is the aspect of TCM that I learned when I studied acupuncture.

For veterinary alternative practitioners, attempting to take the pulse on the radial artery of our patients can be problematic. Fortunately, I discovered how to apply the technique of *surrogate* pulse diagnosis. Adapting the techniques of kinesiology, which recognizes that the energy of the practitioner can merge with that of the patient, I found that if I took my own pulse at the relative positions described above and, at the same moment, contacted the etheric energy of the patient, my pulse would temporarily take on the relative deficiencies and excesses of the animal being examined.

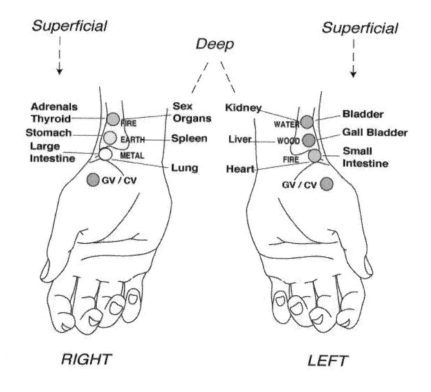

Positions of the organ/meridians on the radial arteries

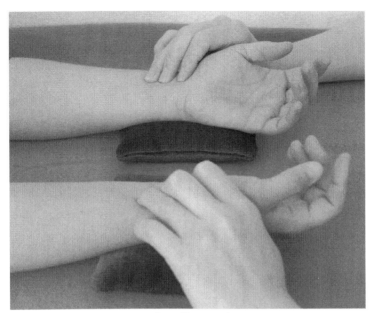

pulse diagnosis

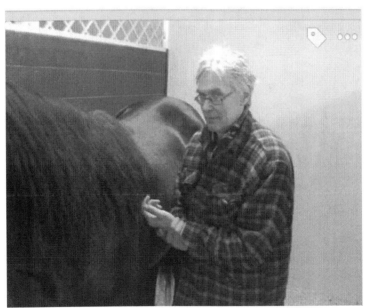

Surrogate Pulse diagnosis

How the Yellow emperor also changed the Pulse-positions to accomplish his deeds.

In hundreds of years before the Yellow Emperor changed the medical system, the Chinese had a 12-element system, where man and woman (Yang and Yin) were separated.
The pulse—diagnosis was also quite different from after the Yellow Emperor.
In creating the 5-elements the main change was that Yin and Yang was put together in the same element, and also both the heart and the pericardium was put together.
This resulted in man and woman was put together, and all differences between them were concealed.
This is, according to Dr. Johannes Weinzirl, leader of the anthroposophic medical courses in Chechia, a main cause of diseases being transferred from parents to children.

This confusion also happened in the 70-ties of the European culture, when the differences between man and woman were obscured, and resulted in massive waves of translocated diseases, such as cancer.

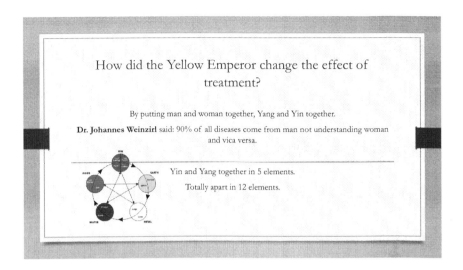

How did the Yellow Emperor change the effect of treatment?

By putting man and woman together, Yang and Yin together.

Dr. Johannes Weinzirl said: 90% of all diseases come from man not understanding woman and vica versa.

Yin and Yang together in 5 elements.

Totally apart in 12 elements.

Also in pulse-diagnosis the same deceit was fulfilled. Before the time of the Yellow Emperor the positions of the Yin and the Yang, the female and the male, were far apart. Now they also were put together at the wrist of the human being, bringing man and woman together as if they were the same, as if they were one, thus preparing for the possibility of translocation.

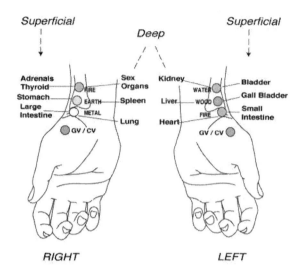

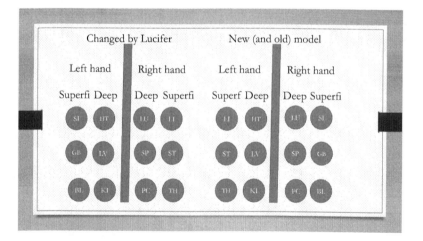

Here we see how the nowadays used system of pulse-diagnosis must be changed in the same way as the 5-elements has to be changed.

In the system that is usually used man and woman are placed together.

This must be changed, so that man is on the other hand of the woman.

In the "new model" we see that all the Yin/Yang pairs are broken up, and that each part of the pair is on the other hand, just as you will later see that we must do to the 5-elements.

The Pulse as an Exercise Toward Spiritual Development.

For those readers versed in these traditional concepts of Chinese Pulse Diagnosis, the description I shall now present regarding pulse diagnosis will appear quite foreign. In my experience, taking the pulse is a precursor for an initiation into the spiritual world. What I am about to teach will be especially useful for those alternative practitioners who are acupuncturists, for this can be their way to access the experience necessary to evoke Christ consciousness.

When I started to teach pulse diagnosis to my students, I thought that it would be easy for them to monitor the pulse diagnostic patterns in their patients. I thought it was a very simple and straight forward method. Therefore, I was astonished when very few were able to master this technique. At the time, I had no explanation for this phenomenon.

I later discovered the reason. The pulse I was feeling was not obtained by my physical senses. The pulse I was looking for was etheric in nature and its true imbalance could only be found by my spiritual senses. My understanding that I always entered the spiritual world when taking a pulse did not come to my conscious attention until much later in life.

Now that we have learned the path to initiation as described by myself and Rudolf Steiner, we can be reminded of the similarities between my path and the method in which I proceed with my diagnostic exam. As I now realize that it is a doorway into the spiritual world, this method will also help us obtain the tools necessary to develop our spiritual organs.

The main skill we must learn is the ability to become detached, to enter a state of not caring, not allowing the mind to wander, and not to act other than taking the pulse.
In this state we start to separate, as described earlier in this book.

In the beginning, the state of indifference can be difficult to obtain. We are often distracted by a wandering or overly concerned mind. Therefore, we should strive to practice our pulse technique in an environment free of emotional obstacles such the judgement of being observed by critical colleagues.

Because we are all anchored to the material world by an entanglement of our thinking, feeling and willing or the fusion of the astral- and etheric bodies, our primary directive must always be in the forefront of our mind, to master the ability to separate the three soul qualities and/or the astral- and etheric bodies.

Our mind may very well influence the result of our diagnostic work, just in the same way that the observer may influence an outcome as stated in quantum physics. Therefore, it is necessary that we maintain a neutral meditative state.[35]

It might also be a help to try to separate the thinking towards the sky, the feeling towards the periphery and the willing towards the earth.

---

[35] The secret life of Plants authored by Tompkins and Bird: The authors discovered that plants respond favorably to the caregiver's positive attitude and negatively to negative emotions.

1. Thinking = height, the upward direction (toward the cosmos).
2. Feeling = width, the outward direction (the expanses of our environment).
3. Willing = depth, the downward direction (as if going into the earth).

Using this information, we can use our imagination and blur the delineation of the three dimensions of our physical world. In other words, we practice "fuzzy vision" by fading away, similar to a day dream where we become unaware of our surroundings as if in the state just before sleep.

Preparation for Taking the Pulse.
Proper pulse taking requires a proper state of mind. This mind set can be described best as a state of day dreaming. When I began to teach the pulse, I urged my students to create the conditions conducive to focused concentration and impartial objectivity. They should create strict rituals. A help in this would be to be immaculately clean and free of physical needs, such as hunger and thirst. The environment required freedom from distractions.

For the beginner, it would help to begin with the preparations that I described above. The first mind set one must adapt is a state of *"not caring"*. Of course, this first sounds as a kind of therapeutic blasphemy, implying an absence of empathy. Quite the contrary, it represents an emphatic thumb's up to faith. It is the opening of a door to the inward stream of information that the Christ impulse brings to us. Thus, the practitioner must not carry preconceptions of the causes of the disease, and shed all interest, anxiety or desire to reach a diagnosis or other prejudicial matter. This stance allows one to live in the exact moment of the pulse and nothing else.

Secondly, along with a sort of indifference, the practitioner must stay focused (*not mind wandering*). One should concentrate totally and exclusively on the patient. The rest of the world has to be blocked out during this procedure.

Finally, the practitioner should *"not act"*. This is actually the description of the achieved meditative state, when one seems to fade away, as if he were under the influence of a hypnotic suggestion. These are the qualities that create the alpha wave activity in the brain to increase. In anthroposophic terms, this is referred to as separating the soul faculties of thinking, feeling and willing[36].

In this state of mind, the separation of the mentioned soul constituents should be easy.

In my experience, the soul faculty of feeling is the simplest to separate. Therefore, one can start the process by separating width from height and depth. I do this by using the tools of anthroposophic meditative techniques to induce a state of daydreaming where one merges into the wide expanses of the surroundings. Imagine yourself listening to a boring lecture. This is the feeling of fading away. When thinking and willing are separated from feeling you feel as if you are floating, and you have no strength nor desire to will or think of anything. Often the sense of hearing will be muted by an internal ringing, and the colours of the landscape will darken, taking on a violet hue. Many find themselves subconsciously tilting their head slightly to the right.

It is now at this point that we direct this separated and pure faculty of feeling to concentrate on the blood flowing in our fingertips from the heart and create a deep connection with our patient and his pulse. It is at this point that we are essentially inside that patient.

While we are learning these techniques, we must also keep in mind the difference between the laws of the physical world and those of the spiritual world. In the spiritual world, we are not

---

[36] Academically, this change between the non-separation and the separation of the soul abilities is called a "noetic slippage". This slippage is a spiritual state where the mind changes between chaos and order, between light and darkness, between Dionysian and apollonian, between the noetic and the chthonic.

bound by dimension and time. With that said, we can travel vast distances in the blink of an eye. We can move through time, as it is no longer absolute. Here a thought becomes an intention and an intention becomes a thing. This is the law of destiny as a reflection of our past and present karma.

As long as we are in the grip of the entanglement of these soul faculties, we cannot detect the energetic changes necessary to truly heal our patients. There are no shortcuts. Despite the descriptive attempts of the use of psychotropic agents by many to induce this state, these methods often create a false presentment of the spiritual world.

The hands as spiritual organs:
Another correlation between Spiritual Science and my development of pulse diagnosis was evident in the lecture given by Rudolf Steiner on August 26, 1912 in Munich. This is what he said regarding the hands as spiritual sense organs:

"The etheric organs of the hands are true spiritual organs. The etheric organs expressed in the hands and their functions, work far more intuitively, more spiritually, and perform a far higher task than is accomplished by the etheric brain. Whoever has made progress in these matters will say that the brain with its etheric basis is in effect by far the least skillful of the spiritual organs man bears within him.

The spiritual activities connected with the organs underlying the hands, but incompletely expressed in the hands and their functions, serve a far higher, more spiritual kind of knowledge and observation. These organs can lead into the super-sensible world and can occupy themselves with our perception and orientation there. A spiritual seer may express this, somewhat surprisingly but accurately, by saying that the human brain is a most clumsy organ for research in the spiritual world, and that the hands, or the spiritual basis of the hands, are far more interesting and significant organs for gaining knowledge of the world, and are certainly far more skillful organs than the brain. Not much is gained on the way to initiation by advancing from the use of the physical brain to a free use of the etheric brain. The difference is not great between what may be achieved through purified, intuitive brain thinking, and regulated spiritual working in the etheric spiritual counterpart of the brain. The difference is much greater between what our hands accomplish in the world, and what can be done by the etheric part that is the spiritual basis of the hands, than the physical brain. On the path of initiation not much development of the etheric brain is necessary, since it is not a particularly important organ. But the etheric basis of the hands is connected with the activity of the lotus flower in the region of the heart, as you will learn in my book; "Knowledge of the Higher Worlds and Its Attainment".

This lotus flower pours out its rays of force in such a way as to build up the organism that, at the stage at which physical man now stands, exists in an incomplete form in the hands and their functions. Though it may sound strange, yet it is true that the least skillful organ for spiritual investigation is the brain, since it is the least capable of development. On the other hand, entirely new perspectives are opened out when we consider other apparently subordinate organs."

From the Head to the Throat to the heart.

As the years passed and my skills intensified, I started to develop my spiritual sense organs. The first spiritual organ was the one of sight. I began to see the etheric energy of myself, my patients, and all living things. I could see it connecting between the trees, then among the animals and among the people.

In the beginning, I felt that my observations originated from the sensory center in the back of the brain, I saw that this energy flowed in a downward direction, traversing my arm, and entering my fingers to act as a source for both diagnosis and healing as I applied the needles to my patients. But then the center where the spiritual observations were made started to wander. First it moved towards the heart, then the spine, and then slowly spread throughout the entire body. The observations also became enlarged from an intellectual observation, to an immediate knowledge of past, present and future from observing what I was feeling from the pulse. The direction of this observation, which now had become knowledge, also changed. In the beginning, the direction of the information streamed from the patient towards me, but then it started to go both ways, as if the patient also received treatment at the same time as I was diagnosing. The observation also enlarged in space, as it also came to include the astral part of the patient's make up. This part was seen as a light flowing area, mingled together with the darker etheric energy. Then the observation started to move in time, to where past, present and future became one.

The first picture shown below, demonstrates what I spiritually see in the head of a beginner taking the pulse. The soul qualities of thinking, feeling and willing are entangled. In this way, the thought processes are consumed with daily living, leaving little etheric energy for pulse diagnosis or treating the patient.

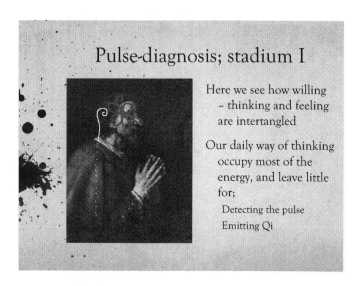

However, with training, years of practice and correct meditation, the soul faculties begin to separate, allowing the stream of energy from the head to strengthen. This ultimately improves the ability of the practitioner to both diagnose and treat.

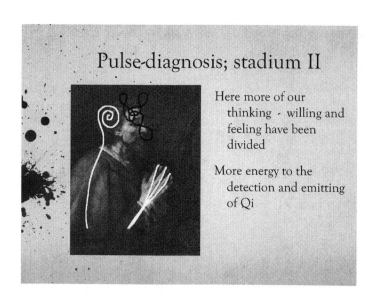

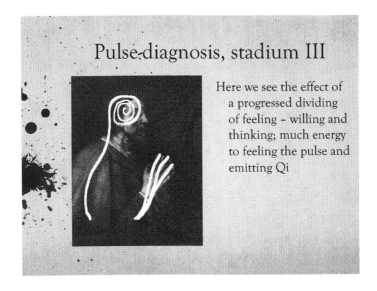

Pulse-diagnosis, stadium III

Here we see the effect of a progressed dividing of feeling – willing and thinking; much energy to feeling the pulse and emitting Qi

As thinking, feeling and willing become disengaged from one another, the etheric energy that is centered in the head begins to move downward. This movement is closely linked to the development of Christianity, when Christ appeared on earth. This is the movement toward the heart.

The 12-petal lotus flower: The etheric Heart Organ.
The lotus flowers of anthroposophy represent the spiritual sense organs of the soul faculties. The twelve-petal lotus, in particular, characterizes the makeup of the heart chakra as the center of selfless love, the residence of the Christ impulse and the eventual source of a vast etheric energy that we can utilize to help our patients. According to Rudolf Steiner, six of these petals already exist in us, while the other six must be developed by ourselves. The 12-petal lotus, when developed, reveals to the budding clairvoyant a deep understanding of the process of nature and the Christ impulse.

Rudolf Steiner says the following about this development.

"When esoteric development has progressed so far that the lotus flowers begin to stir, much has already been achieved by the student which can result in the formation of certain quite definite currents and movements in his etheric body. The object of this development is the formation of a kind of center in the region of the physical heart, from which radiate currents and movements in the greatest possible variety of colours and forms. The center is in reality not a mere point, but a most complicated structure, a most wonderful organ. It glows and shimmers with every shade of colours and displays forms of great symmetry, capable of rapid transformation. Other forms and streams of colours radiate from this organ to the other parts of the body, and beyond it to the astral body, completely penetrating and illuminating it. The most important of these currents flow to the lotus flowers. They permeate each petal and regulate its revolutions; then streaming out at the points of the petals, they lose themselves in outer space. The higher the development of a person, the greater the circumference to which these rays extend.*
The twelve-petal lotus flower has a particularly close connection with this central organ. The currents flow directly into it and through it, proceeding on the one side to the sixteen and the two-petal lotus flowers, and on the other, the lower side, to the flowers of eight, six and four petals. It is for this reason that the very greatest care must be devoted to the development of the twelve-petal lotus, for an imperfection in the latter would result in irregular formation of the whole structure. The above will give an idea of the delicate and intimate nature of esoteric training, and of the accuracy needed if the development is to be regular and correct. It will also be evident beyond doubt that directions for the development of super sensible faculties can only be the concern of those who have*

themselves experienced everything which they propose to awaken in others, and who are unquestionably in a position to know whether the directions they give lead to the exact results desired. If the student follows the directions that have been given him, he introduces into his etheric body currents and movements which are in harmony with the laws and the evolution of the world to which he belongs. Consequently, these instructions are reflections of the great laws of cosmic evolution. They consist of the above-mentioned and similar exercises in meditation and concentration, which, if correctly practiced, produce the results described. The student must at certain times let these instructions permeate his soul with their content, so that he is inwardly entirely filled with it. A simple start is made with a view to the deepening of the logical activity of the mind and the producing of an inward intensification of thought. Thought is thereby made free and independent of all sense impressions and experiences; it is concentrated in one point, which is held entirely under control. Thus, a preliminary center is formed for the currents of the etheric body. This center is not yet in the region of the heart but in the head, and it appears to the clairvoyant as the point of departure for movements and currents. No esoteric training can be successful which does not first create this center. If the latter were first formed in the region of the heart the aspiring clairvoyant would doubtless obtain glimpses of the higher worlds, but would lack all true insight into the connection between these higher worlds and the world of our senses. This, however, is an unconditional necessity for man at the present stage of evolution. The clairvoyant must not become a visionary; he must retain a firm footing upon the earth. The center in the head, once duly fixed, is then moved lower down, to the region of the larynx. This is affected by further exercises in concentration. Then the currents of the etheric body radiate from this point and illuminate the astral space surrounding the individual.

Continued practice enables the student to determine for himself the position of this etheric body. Hitherto this position depends upon external forces proceeding from the physical body. Through further development the student is able to turn his etheric body to all sides. This faculty is effected by currents moving approximately along both hands and centered in the two-petal lotus in the region of the eyes. All this is made possible through the radiations from the larynx assuming round forms, of which a number flow to the two-petal lotus and thence form undulating currents along the hands. As a further development, these currents branch out and ramify in the most delicate manner and become, as it were, a kind of web which then encompasses the entire etheric body as though with a network. Whereas hitherto the etheric body was not closed to the outer world, so that the life currents from the universal ocean of life flowed freely in and out, these currents now have to pass through this membrane. Thus, the individual becomes sensitive to these external streams; they become perceptible to him.

And now the time has come to give the complete system of currents and movements its center situated in the region of the heart. This again is affected by persevering with the exercises in concentration and meditation; and at this point also the stage is reached when the student becomes gifted with the inner word. All things now acquire a new significance for him. They become as it were, spiritually audible in their innermost self, and speak to him of their essential being. The currents described above place him in touch with the inner being of the world to which he belongs. He begins to mingle his life with the life of his environment and can let it reverberate in the movements of his lotus flowers."

Concentration on the heart.

Before I take the pulse, I begin by separating and isolating the soul faculty of "feeling". I discard my own ego-centered feelings, and replace them with a global love for everything. Later, when I consider the diagnosis (thinking) and treatment (willing), I also leave the other two faculties, either feeling and willing or thinking and feeling, and try to use only one of the divine forces.

However, when I first enter the diagnostic process, I enter my feeling force through my own heart, and concentrate on the heart of the patient. I visualize that I am creating a tunnel or portal between my own heart and that of the patient. I enter this tunnel only with my feeling, leaving both the thinking and the willing outside. In going towards the heart of the patient, I now imagine the 12-layer microsystem of sheaths that begins at the physical skin of the patient and ends in the inside of his spiritual heart.

I first picture going through the 8 layers of the body of the patient, and then into the 4 layers of the heart, a total of 12 layers. The 8th layer is where we move past the body to enter the 9th layer, represented by the endocardium, and enter the realm of the heart, the spiritual center of man. In this moment we go from the material realm of the body and into the spiritual realm of the heart.

Most students stop before the 8th layer, and are unable to enter the heart. It appears that this step requires the presence of a strong and determined will in order to push past this level. It is easiest to understand how to accomplish this if we first learn to visualize these 12 layers of the body as listed below

1. The outer layer (1) relate to the physical body.
2. The next (2rd) to the astral body.
3. The 3rd to the etheric body.

4. The 4th parasitic bodies. Note that the parasites situate themselves close to the life-energy of the physical body, between the etheric body and the life-ether.

5. The 5th-6th-7th-8th relate to the 4 ethers.

   a. 5th - life ether.

   b. 6th - chemical ether.

   c. 7th - light ether.

   d. 8th - warmth-ether, touching the pericardium, where we leave the material world, and in the 9th layer we enter the spiritual world-

6. The inner layers (9th-10th-11th-12th) are within the heart, and relate to the "I"; the lower I (9th), the middle I (10th), the higher I (11th) and the cosmic I (the Christ consciousness) (12th), where we are in the middle of the heart, the lamb (ram), the Christ consciousness.

When we are in the middle of the heart, we should imagine standing at a cross. This cross is a little different in a man, a horse and a dog.

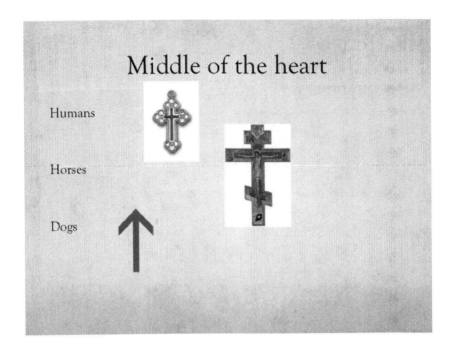

Middle of the heart

Humans

Horses

Dogs

On the way through the 12 layers we may diagnose, experience and/or treat the different aspects present in these layers concerning diseases or spiritual realities. For example, the two outer layers relate to the astral body of the patient. These layers reflect feelings and emotions. If we stop at this layer, and take the pulse here, we get an emotional diagnosis.

The 3rd and 4th layers both reflect the physical body. The third layer being our own physical body and the fourth related to the material bodies of parasites that exist within us. If we stop evaluating the pulse at the 3rd or 4th layer we will be able to diagnose the imbalances present in the physical body. Exploring the pulse at the 4th layer is especially interesting as here we can detect the presence of both physical and energetic parasites in the body of the patient.

The layers where most beginners seem to stop is at the etheric level, located between the 5th and the 8th layer. This is the location of healing energy of the life force that can be activated by acupuncture and homeopathy.

Between the 8th and the 9th layer lies the departure from the physical aspects of the body and the beginning of the spiritual heart organ. I discovered that this region is useful to diagnose the presence of a blockage created by a toxic scar. These particular scars can prevent a successful treatment. I found that when there is no deficiency in the 8th layer, and a clear deficiency in the 9th layer, a blocking scar is present. I then focus my intention while taking the pulse at this level to *find* the exact location of the scar, but later realized that it is possible to just *treat* them using the pulse findings at the 12th layer. Earlier in my career, when I found them I would inject them with procaine, as described in neural therapy by Dr. Ferdinand Hünecke.[37] I now find this to be unnecessary, as I have learned to always treat using the findings when focused on the 12th layer.

I feel that the four layers within the heart itself are of immense importance. From here we may diagnose and treat diseases from

---

[37] The father of neural therapy: The idea underlying the therapy is that "interference fields" (*Störfelder*) at certain sites of the body are responsible for a type of electric energy that causes illness. The fields can be disrupted by injection, allowing the body to heal. The practice originated in 1925 when Ferdinand Hünecke, a German surgeon, used a newly launched pain drug that contained procaine (a local anaesthetic) on his sister who had severe intractable migraines. Instead of using it intramuscularly as recommended he injected it intravenously and the migraine attack stopped immediately. He and his brother Walter subsequently used Novocaine in a similar way to treat a variety of ailments. In 1940 Ferdinand Hüneke injected the painful shoulder of a woman who also had an osteomyelitis in her leg, which at that time (before antibiotics) threatened her with amputation. The shoulder pain improved somewhat but the leg wound became itchy. On injecting the leg wound the shoulder pain vanished immediately – a reaction he called the "phenomenon of seconds" (*Sekundenphänomen*).

the spiritual realm of the patient. This, in my opinion is the best option to cure the patient

The inner (9th - 10th - 11th - 12th) are within the heart, and relate to the "I"; the lower I (9th), the middle I (10th), the higher I (11th) and the cosmic I (the Christ consciousness) (12th), where we are in the middle of the heart, where the lamb (ram), the Christ consciousness resides. When we treat from the middle of the heart, we are in the deepest spiritual realm, and here the usual stumbling blocks are gone.

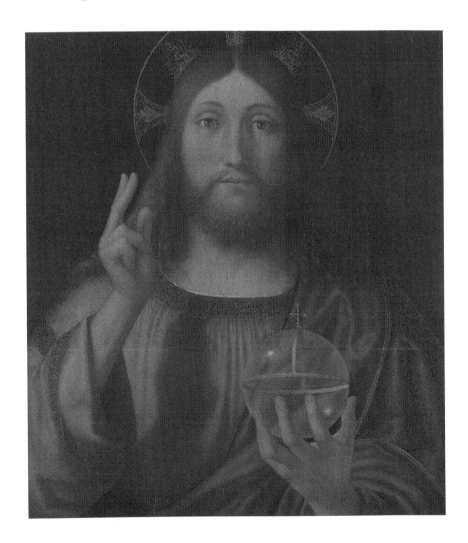

How to practice transformation or translocation from our minds, schematically.

Now we will describe schematically how to use our **mind** to **perform** these tasks.

1. First go into the calm non-caring, no-wanting and no-doing mood.
2. Separate one or more soul-properties or spiritual parts, especially the etheric from the astral or the thinking from the feeling or the feeling from the willing.
3. Pass the Threshold.
4. Activate one or more of the spiritual sense-organs. Personally, I always use the eyes, situated within the physical eyes, not behind and not in front.
5. Observe spiritually the spiritual constituents of the patient, the electro-magnetic devise or the area containing earth-radiation. For this I usually use a combination of the heart and feeling in connection with the eyes, clairvoyance.
6. While observing the adversarial components of the items in question, activate you will-power. To do this you have to separate the will from the rest of the body.
7. Let the will stream downwards into the earth, followed by an upstreaming.
8. Meet the upstreaming will-force with the intention-impregnated thinking, which may be called intention, and let a union of these two streams flow towards the adversarial forces, the earth radiation or the observed demon, and just kindly lead them away, which will be a translocation.
9. Another possibility is the push the two adversarial forces apart, as there always are two forces, one distal and one proximal. In this pushing away give room for the entering of the Christ force, the Christ-consciousness.

10. In leading them away (translocation), or in starting a transformation in the name of Christ, also fill your soul with a compassion and mood of asking excuse for having made the divine powers into adversarial beings by our deeds.

A person that was able to master both Translocation and Transformation; Anna Katerina Emmerick.

Blessed Anne Catherine Emmerich (also *Anna Katharina Emmerick*; born on the 8th of September 1774 – dead on the 9th of February 1824) was a Roman Catholic Augustinian Canoness Regular of Windesheim, mystic, Marian visionary, ecstatic and stigmatist.

She was born in Flamschen, a farming community at Coesfeld, in the Diocese of Münster, Westphalia, Germany, and died at age 49 in Dülmen, where she had been a nun, and later become bedridden. Emmerich experienced visions on the life and passion of Jesus Christ, reputed to be revealed to her by the Blessed Virgin Mary under religious ecstasy.

During her bedridden years, a number of well-known figures were inspired to visit her. The poet Clemens Brentano interviewed her at length and wrote two books based on his notes of her visions. The authenticity of Brentano's writings has been questioned and critics have characterized the books as "conscious elaborations by a poet" and a "well-intentioned fraud" by Brentano.

Emmerich was beatified on 3 October 2004, by Pope John Paul II. However, the Vatican focused on her own personal piety rather than the religious writings associated to her by Clemens Brentano.

This nun was able to, by will, translocate all different diseases that her visitors had, onto herself, and then, during 2-3 days to transform then.

This transformation was always painful to her, and she suffered a great deal in this process.

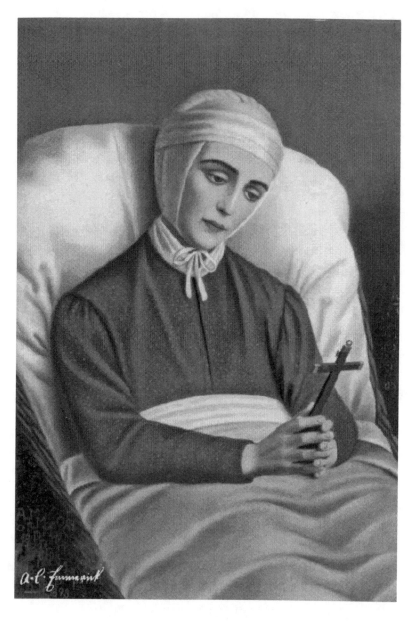

Anna Katerina Emmerich (1774 – 1824)

On the back side of the book

This book is about translocation within acupuncture.

Separation can occur with the adversarial forces that cause disease, and this is called 'translocation'.

Translocation is often caused by the application of natural healing methods as acupuncture.

Understanding and using the 7 or 12 elements, the middle-point or Christ-force can hinder translocation and further a transformation of the adversarial forces.

In this was we can give our patients a true healing.

Made in the USA
Middletown, DE
27 October 2020